Everything
I know
about
hormones.

Everything I know about hormones.

SIX STEPS TO OPTIMAL HEALTH & HAPPINESS

Hannah Alderson

BANT-registered nutritionist

DK
[RED]

3. The Positive Method 116

Introduction

As I sit here, I feel incredibly lucky. I've worked hard on my hormones, health, happiness, and career. But, like most things, there was a dash of luck involved. I was lucky enough to trust my gut and ask more questions, not taking "no" for an answer when doctors brushed me off. I was lucky enough to have private healthcare, a supportive family, and access to education, which helped me pivot my career and take my wellness into my own hands. I am now lucky to live symptom-free with two beautiful children, Otis and Dusty – something I once thought impossible. I am lucky to support women daily in my clinic – women who were once lost and overwhelmed like me.

The best luck of all, though, is sharing everything I know about hormones and sprinkling a little luck your way, too.

It's a privilege to reflect on my hormone story as I write this. I'm not going to lie; it's been a wild ride. As many readers will know first-hand, hormones don't always follow the script.

MY HORMONE STORY

Throughout my teenage years, my periods were often irregular and painful. Back in the '90s and early 2000s, going on the pill was the norm and, like most kids my age, I started taking an oral contraception pill at age 16. It was a disaster for me, negatively impacting my weight and mental health, and leading me to suffer from terrible mood swings. I was then put onto a different oral contraceptive that I continued to take for several years.

I grew up during a horrendous era for diet culture and body image. My toes still curl when I remember walking into my first diet club meeting at 16 with my mum, held in an echoey village hall where nutritional advice was being dished out as quickly as the branded diet bars.

This was where my journey with yo-yo dieting began, driven by a constantly fluctuating weight due to a condition called polycystic ovarian syndrome, or PCOS. Despite exhibiting all the most common symptoms at the time, I didn't know that I had PCOS and wouldn't receive my diagnosis until five years later.

As my weight fluctuated ever more dramatically during my late teens, my preoccupation with dieting deepened. My changing body shape, mixed with feelings of anxiety and erratic cycles or unusually long periods, made me feel low, lost, and lacklustre. I couldn't understand what was wrong.

In my early twenties, I finally decided to come off the pill. However, my period didn't reappear. My doctor told me this was nothing to worry about but, a year and a half later, it still hadn't returned, and with continued weight changes and congested skin, my feelings of anxiety were crippling.

I could not understand why my body felt so unstable. Why did I suddenly become short of breath in mildly stressful scenarios? Why did I catastrophize the small things? Why did my excess weight centre around my middle? Why was I constantly tired? Why was my skin so inflamed and spotty? Outwardly, I presented as being a bright and popular drama scholar, who went on to get a First-Class Degree and a Royal National Theatre Student Award. But underneath it all, I felt like a failure. Was I failing at being a woman because I wasn't having periods? Was I failing at being desirable as I wasn't thinner? The sad thing is, I was never actually overweight. I was just a young woman trying to keep up with unrealistic beauty standards. Sadly, I know so many women have been made to feel the same.

At age 21, a doctor mentioned PCOS to me. I'd never heard of this condition, and it wasn't until a few years later that I was officially diagnosed, after a routine smear revealed abnormal cells in my cervix. My periods still hadn't returned after stopping the pill, so while having these abnormal cells removed, I negotiated

PCOS

PCOS is an endocrine disorder driven by an imbalance of hormones, typically producing excessive amounts of testosterone, cortisol, and insulin. A collection of specific symptoms unique to each individual, PCOS can be linked to insulin resistance, inflammation, and high stress. Symptoms often include irregular or absent periods, fluctuations in weight, anxiety, fatigue, excess hair growth, sleep issues, and skin conditions.

getting an internal scan of my ovaries. The scan, along with further blood tests, confirmed the diagnosis of PCOS. No one explained it to me. Like so many women, I was left to face it alone.

Back then, I didn't realize that PCOS is one of the most common yet frequently undiagnosed conditions affecting women. Globally, it's estimated to affect 8–13 per cent of women. Still, according to the World Health Organization, up to 70 per cent of women with PCOS remain undiagnosed.

After being told I had PCOS, the advice was to either go back on the pill or wait until I wanted children, at which point I could start taking metformin (a medication for type 2 diabetes) or clomiphene (a drug that stimulates ovulation in women). The word "infertility" was thrown around, taking root in my already anxious subconscious. Was I going to fail at motherhood, too? I took the advice, confident that medical professionals knew best, and decided to wait it out until I wanted to start a family.

In a bid to manage my yo-yoing weight, I jumped between fad diets and juice cleanses. But eating less and exercising more won't solve any underlying metabolic issues. When your metabolic profile causes your body to prioritize the accumulation of fat, even your best efforts may leave you feeling frustrated. The elevated levels of insulin and cortisol associated with PCOS, for instance, can make conventional advice from your doctor less helpful. I have worked with hundreds of women who have been failed by a medical system that does not understand the complexities of this disorder.

I tried everything – the Special K challenge, Atkins, Dukan, the apple diet, the maple syrup fast and, for a long stint when I was living in New York and trying to make it onto Broadway, I took up veganism after reading *Skinny Bitch*. At the turn of the millennium, I was living life fast and dirty; hydration was based on Diet Coke, sleep was in short supply, my diet was poor, and my beauty regime consisted of face wipes.

Little did I know that this kind of inflammatory lifestyle, paired with terrible sleep patterns and high stress, would drive my hormonal imbalance and worsen another condition I later found out I had – endometriosis. At 26, I had started experiencing serious pain in my lower abdomen. It was a scratching, aching pain that seemed to radiate from both ovaries. I'd recently had the copper

ENDOMETRIOSIS

Endometriosis is an oestrogen-dependent inflammatory condition that occurs when tissue similar to the lining of the uterus grows outside of the uterus. Think of it like a period bleed happening in your body but with nowhere to go, so painful and inflamed lesions form.

coil fitted – having been told this was a better choice for me than the pill, as it was hormone-free – and assumed that this was the cause. I was also feeling even more tired, but put it down to all the late nights on the town, living my best life like any girl in her twenties.

I tried to ignore my symptoms, until one day the pain was so intense that I couldn't leave the house. It was engulfing and ferocious, like metal scraping across soft, tender tissue, radiating from my core like a throbbing earthquake. The only thing that comes close to a comparison is childbirth. Sex was painful. Going to the loo was painful. It was a lot!

With conditions like endometriosis, you can't see the source of pain. And if you can't see it, is it even there? I was made to feel like I was imagining things, something I continue to hear about from clients all too frequently. Doctors told me that I had "trapped wind", and I was instructed once again to "eat less", "move more", and "lose weight" as a way of solving my PCOS. At one point, I was even offered antidepressants – and this was not the issue. I was being brushed off and gaslit. I felt overwhelmed, let down by the system and desperately worried that I would never become a mother. Something had to change.

TAKING CONTROL

At this point, aged 27, I embarked on a journey of discovery – and self-initiated research.

I started to frequent healthcare shops, searching for supplements that might help my PCOS. What could this tea do? What benefits might the *Vitex* plant have? Should I be taking inositol? I could spend hours in these shops, with their calming magical treasure troves of powders and herbs. This was before social media as we know it today, where most women now turn to for wellness advice, so it felt very lonely. But it was within these healthcare shops that I felt like I was onto something. I consulted a homeopath. Though I realized homeopathy wasn't for me, she got me thinking about food and nutrition. I devoured Alisa Vitti's book *WomanCode*, and tuned into the BBC Radio 4 Food Programme. After discovering the work of integrative gynaecologist and PCOS expert Dr Felice Gersh, I began researching the link between diet and PCOS. For the first time, I started to understand what PCOS actually was.

I took up running, quit Diet Coke, and started making smoothies in the morning instead of skipping breakfast, all of which did wonders for my mental health and energy levels.

Meanwhile, I was inspired by people like Madeleine Shaw and Ella Woodward of Deliciously Ella, who were making waves in the wellness scene. I started a blog, and it felt like flicking on a switch. Soon after this, my mum asked me over lunch, "Why don't you follow this passion and study nutrition?"

I realized that this was the path I needed to follow to be the best version of me, and help support women in similar situations. This wish led me to train as a BANT-registered nutritionist and then as a functional medicine practitioner.

What followed would be a deep understanding of how nutrition, lifestyle, and a positive mindset are all integral to supporting your hormone health. I began implementing dietary changes, running functional tests on myself, and creating my own supplement plan. My period returned, and it was regular.

At the age of 30, I ignored all those years of medical gaslighting and took my pain to a specialist in London, Dr Colin Davis. He really listened to me and, in doing so, changed my life. Following surgery, I finally received a formal diagnosis: I had severe stage 4 endometriosis. I had lesions around my fallopian tubes, ovaries, and "pouch of Douglas" – the area between the uterus and the rectum.

After surgery, both my endometriosis and PCOS symptoms gradually diminished, aided by lifestyle and dietary changes like switching to blood sugar-balancing whole foods instead of ultra-processed foods, and incorporating nurturing exercise instead of intense cardio workouts. I embraced the positive practices of self-love and creativity.

LOOKING AHEAD

My mission now is to educate and empower. For the last seven years, I've run a private practice specializing in women's health and supporting women across the globe. I provide women with the knowledge needed to navigate hormonal health and happiness through nutrition, sleep, movement, self-love, a positive mindset, and creativity.

I wrote this book to equip you with holistic tools to manage your hormonal health. It's not just for those who suffer from hormone-related conditions like PCOS and endometriosis. If you have ever struggled to understand what is going on inside your own body, if you have "battled through" the pain because you didn't think it was worth speaking up, or if you have ever been dismissed by doctors or medical professionals, this book is for you. I want you to know that I have been in your shoes – and you have the power to create a brighter future.

These days, we have a better understanding of how hormones affect women at almost every life stage – from the first period to fertility, menopause, and beyond. We know that teenage girls are more likely to be affected by anxiety. We know about the hormone rollercoaster for new mothers and their increased risk of depression. We are learning how to adapt our movement to our menstrual cycles. There's now much more discussion about perimenopause and menopause, along with improved access to hormone replacement therapies. The world is changing, and hormones are beginning to receive the attention they deserve.

Despite this progress, hormone health is still often misunderstood and dismissed, and the internet is full of conflicting information.

This book is your one-stop guide for all things hormones – whether you're a teenager riding the waves of puberty, whether you're thinking about having a baby, or whether you're navigating the menopause years. The more knowledge you have, the better equipped you will be to make choices that improve your health – and, in doing so, improve your life.

Getting a handle on your hormones can be simple, affordable and – dare I say it – even *fun*.

So strap in, ladies. Let's begin.

1.

The Landscape of Changing Hormones

The Hormone Crisis

The landscape of women's health is changing. Obesity is at an all-time high, and our little women are reaching puberty at a younger age. Cancer and infertility rates are rising among younger women, and research shows menopause symptoms are starting earlier and becoming more severe. Microplastics, which disrupt hormone balance by mimicking or blocking hormones, have been found in human hearts and placentas. Today, hormone balance is increasingly compromised.

Our hormones and DNA haven't mutated over the decades – but the world has. Diet, lifestyle, big food corporations, big farming, toxins, plastics, pandemics, technology, smartphones, and stress levels – it's a hard place for your hormones to live. Exhaustion is glorified over rest while ever-increasing work hours, addictive smartphones, ultra-processed foods, microplastics, and unsafe tap water combine to create a toxic melting pot. The world is different today than it was 50 years ago – let alone millions of years ago, when the blueprint for our hormone function was set. Every woman should be armed with the tools to give your hormones a helping hand.

A LEGACY OF BLAMING HORMONES

Being "hormonal" isn't usually a compliment; we are quick to blame our hormones for nearly everything. Where has this negativity come from?

History is awash with tales of hormonal hysteria. The term "hormone" was coined over a century ago. Before that, the inner workings of the female endocrine system have been debated upon and theorized at length, mainly by men using fairly unscientific methods, with an emphasis placed on emotional causes – not biological ones. According to the ancient Egyptians, irrational behaviour in females was caused by the spontaneous movement of their uterus. The Greeks would follow this up with more tales of women's madness, attributing hysteria to an "unhappy" womb deprived of sexual activity and childrearing. They declared the cure to be catharsis through wine orgies (led by a male priest. Of course.).

After centuries of shame-inducing labels like "hysterical" and "hormonal", seeking help for "women's problems" often results in doors being slammed in our faces faster than you can say "witch". There is a generational instinct to blame and shame our hormones, an unconscious bias against our amazing biology.

This stops here: your hormones are not to blame. You're about to learn just how incredible they truly are. Hormones are your superpower, and your female biology is something to be proud of. You've just got to work with them, not against them.

THE BRUSH OFF

With inadequate support for hormonal symptoms and even medical gaslighting, many of us feel like our health concerns are being brushed off. Beneath this, there is a thirst for knowledge and a longing for guidance – and women are looking to social media for health advice. Research from the US, China, UK, Germany and Japan found that 33 per cent of GenZ, 26 per cent of millennials, 14 per cent of GenX, and 5 per cent of baby boomers use social media to find support and discuss illness.

A UK government Women's Health Strategy Report highlighted the obstacles women face in getting the care they need, stating that 4 in 5 women felt their healthcare professionals were not listening to them, with 84 per cent of women reporting that there have been times when they, or a woman they knew, were not listened to by healthcare professionals. Additionally, a report from the University of York highlighted the results of women's symptoms not being taken seriously, with significant delays to addressing hormonal disorders and broader menstrual health issues. Women over the age of 65 remarked on feeling "invisible".

Globally, conditions like endometriosis take an average of 6.6 years to be diagnosed. Women with endometriosis say they feel "gaslit" by doctors, while those with PCOS are frustrated by the lack of involvement from medical practitioners and information available. Millions of women around the world are entering menopause without the support they need.

In my clinic, the majority of my clients tell me they have felt let down, lost, or overwhelmed about their hormonal health.

Pointing fingers at failing healthcare systems won't solve much, though. The lack of funding and research into women's health is clear, and I don't blame doctors for it. Where I'm based in the UK, the tremendous pressure on doctors has only continued to snowball since COVID-19. This isn't just a UK-specific problem, either – around the world, women repeatedly face a system rigged against their health, rooted in a design created by men for men.

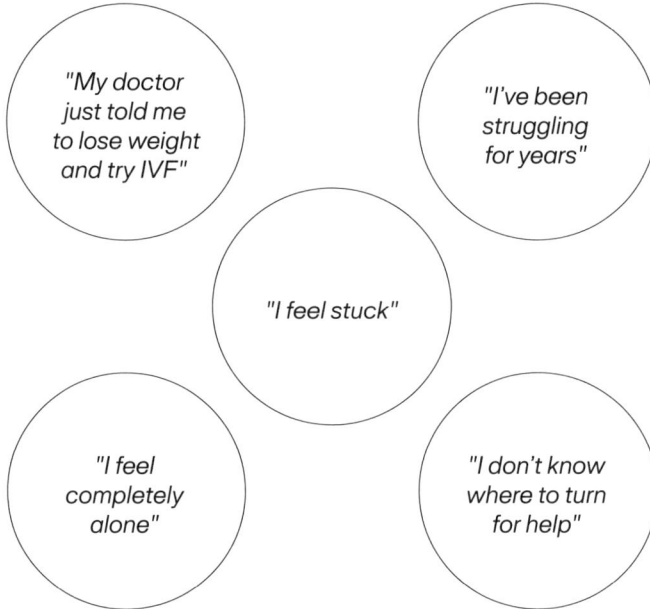

"My doctor just told me to lose weight and try IVF"

"I've been struggling for years"

"I feel stuck"

"I feel completely alone"

"I don't know where to turn for help"

A NEW ERA FOR HORMONE HEALTH

Still, change is afoot. The last few years have seen women-led movements emerge, addressing the gender pay gap and gender pain gap, flexible working hours, and menopause awareness in the workplace, giving heartening signs that a positive shift for women's health may be on the horizon. We might even be on the brink of a generational shift; millennial women are proactively entering perimenopause by planning for "millenopause". Women are asking more questions and taking action, but we still have work to do.

According to the Global Women's Health Index report, "women are more stressed, worried, angry, and sad than at any point in the past decade". The pandemic had a significant emotional impact on female stress and mental health. A 2022 study called The Female Happiness Paradox found that men are generally happier than women and that COVID negatively impacted women's happiness more than men's, based on data from the UK, US, and Europe.

However, the study also discovered that women showed greater resilience during the pandemic – their happiness rebounded more quickly after COVID than men. If women are unhappy but capable of resilience, imagine if they were given the right tools to create happier, healthier lives.

Despite all this, our current climate has created a perfect storm for hormone imbalance via stress, hormone-disrupting chemicals, gender gaps in care and research, misinformation, social pressure, ultra-processed food, and sedentary lifestyles.

Evidence shows that the average age of puberty in girls has dropped by about three months per decade since the 1970s, while PCOS is becoming a significant public health concern with rates increasing around the world at an alarming rate. Cases of early-onset menopause are being linked to hormone-disrupting chemicals in flame retardants and rising rates of obesity. Fertility rates have declined, aligning with a global slowdown in population growth.

Of course, fertility rates are multifactorial, with numerous social and economic factors at play alongside the changing landscape of hormones, from economic insecurity and employment pressures, access to contraception, and the age of first-time pregnancy being higher than in previous generations. These are complex statistics, but it's logical to propose the rise of female endocrine disorders and declining sperm rates (it takes two to tango) have their part to play.

More research is needed to show how toxins, pesticides, mould, and other endocrine-disrupting agents affect our hormonal balance. Instead of hiding from the storm, it's time we face it. We can't necessarily change the weather, but we can learn how to prepare for it.

HORMONAL HEALTH
Optimal hormonal health and wellbeing can
be nurtured from balancing food, movement,
sleep, and positivity.

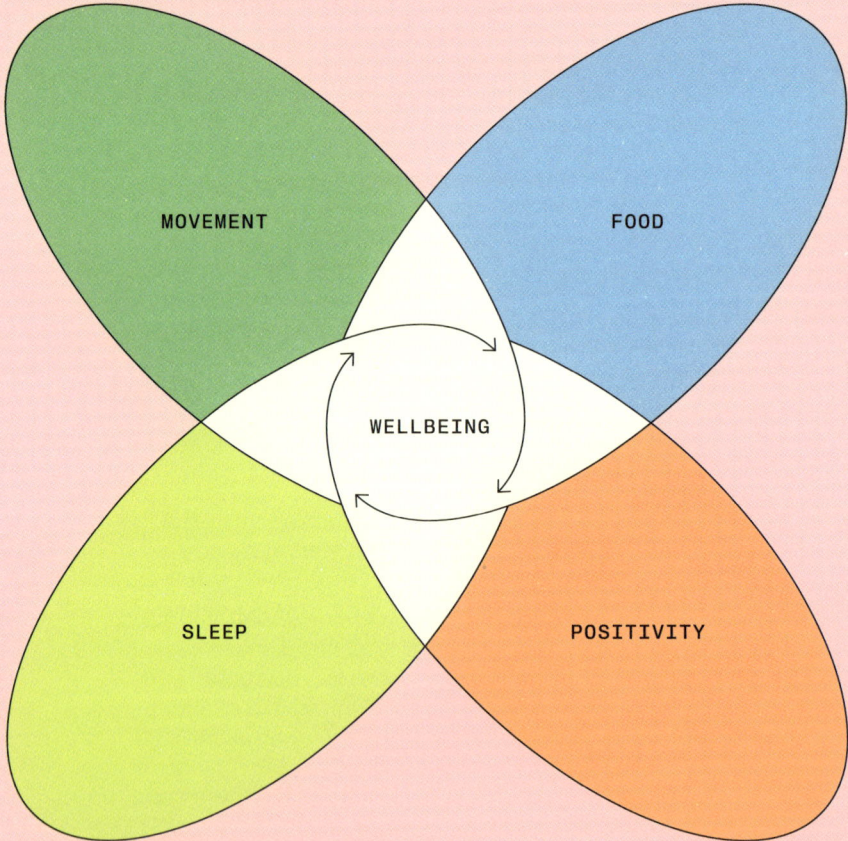

CHARTING THE COURSE

The approach we take to hormonal health must evolve with this changing landscape. We must share our stories to educate, empower, and change the narrative as a community. These pages contain everything I have learned in my health journey – both personal and professional. I use the most recent scientific research to empower women to take control of their hormonal health.

Every facet of our lives impacts how our bodies function. Each of these is an important tool.

FOOD
MOVEMENT
SLEEP
POSITIVITY

Proper nutrition, healthy movement, quality sleep, and a positive mindset can change your hormonal picture and environment. Through my clients, I've learned that our bodies communicate with us, crying out daily with signs and symptoms when they are unhappy. I will teach you how to listen and how to respond.

In exchange, I ask you to shift your focus from frustration – whether it's your hormones, the healthcare system, or corrupt corporations – and instead focus on the steps you can take for a happier, healthier future. This is a chance for positive change that we can navigate together.

The best is yet to come.

2.

The House of Hormones

Harmonizing With Your Hormones

Your hormones are the drivers and distributors of your energy, sleep, mood, waistline, libido, and overall wellbeing. They protect you and help to create life, keeping your heart beating while shaping the bond between a newborn and a parent, fostering the greatest thing on earth – love.

So, where can it all go wrong?

At our core, we are biological machines hardwired to survive. Your body works to protect you and is one of the most amazing biological systems on the planet, thanks to evolution and your survival optimization system.

Managing your hormones is no mean feat. Keeping order requires careful balancing, with all parties highly sensitive to their environment. Working together, your hormones carry out an intricate dance that we call your endocrine system. Hormone balance can collapse like a row of dominoes; when one goes, all the rest can come crashing down. Two hormones in particular, cortisol and insulin, dominate the rest when it comes to impacting other hormones.

Cortisol, produced by the adrenal glands, is your main stress hormone and involved in your sleep–wake cycle, metabolism, and immune response. Insulin, produced by the pancreas, regulates your blood sugar. As you foster a hormone-friendly home, much of your effort will be focused on creating balance between these two hormones.

If you're reading this and have previously felt overwhelmed by all the information out there, or simply just stuck, you're in the right place. You might have felt like your hormones weren't listening, or that they've caused you nothing but misery and frustration. But it's important to realize that, ultimately, they've got your back. Your hormones are, in fact, in your corner.

The trick is to work with them, not against them. Like characters in the screenplay of your life – each one plays a role that can be influenced by you.

LET'S MEET THE FAMILY

There are over 50 hormones in the human body. Do you need to know them all? No, is the short answer. We are going to work from a need-to-know basis, because life is too short to count calories, iron bed linen or understand every single hormone in the human body. Below is a slimmed-down list to keep things fresh and focused.

You'll meet a sprinkling of other hormones along the way, bringing clarity to the complexities of hormone health and how to navigate it.

CORTISOL A steroid stress hormone	**INSULIN** Your glucose regulator
OXYTOCIN Your love hormone	**MELATONIN** Your sleep hormone
SEROTONIN Your happy neurotransmitter	**THYROID HORMONES** Your metabolic regulators impacting energy, growth, and metabolism
OESTROGEN, PROGESTERONE, TESTOSTERONE Your sexual characteristic and reproductive hormones	**FSH AND LSH** Your follicle stimulator (FSH) and your ovulation trigger (LSH)

HORMONE SENSITIVITY

Some hormones are more sensitive than others. Your male sexual characteristic hormones, for instance, are generally more robust, while your female sexual characteristic hormones are more prone to disruption. Think of the care needed when handling cashmere versus cotton – cashmere requires delicate handling, while cotton can withstand more wear and tear.

When oestrogen is not behaving as it should, it can manifest as irregular or heavy periods, weight gain, breast tenderness, histamine intolerance, bloating, or headaches. If your thyroid is dysregulated, symptoms include weight gain, fatigue, brittle hair, sensitivity to the cold, heart palpitations, aching muscles, and constipation. Meanwhile, if your progesterone is out of whack, you might experience high levels of anxiety, a low libido, shorter and lighter periods, spotting, hot flushes, or disrupted sleep.

Your hormones are dedicated to supporting your optimal health, but modern diets and lifestyles can sometimes harm this balance (see pp.107–08), so it's essential to prioritize proper care and awareness to maintain hormonal health.

Every facet of your life has an impact on your body. Your hormones require specific nutrients for their production, optimal function and maintenance. Food plays a powerful role in this process, and your nutritional intake has the power to change your hormonal picture – along with your sleep, movement, and positivity – and everything you absorb and surround yourself with.

When something is going wrong, your hormones will get loud, turning up the volume and affecting everything from your mood to your sleep schedule. Remember, first and foremost, that they are messengers. Tune in to whatever hormonal symptoms are most prominent for you right now.

HORMONE BALANCE – NOT METRICS

Your body is talking to you all the time. From the many hundreds of clients who I have had the pleasure of working with, I see first-hand how women's bodies communicate, especially when they are crying out with daily signs and symptoms that they are not happy. I want to teach you how to listen, and how to respond.

....
What clues is your body giving to you right now?
....
What about over this last week?
....
Why did you pick up this book?
....

This is a good time for you to get grounded, and "check in" by putting pen to paper. One way to do this is with the MYMOP (Measure Yourself Medical Outcome Profile) tool, which I use in clinic with my clients (see overleaf, pp.26–27).

This is a time stamp of your symptoms, and one that you can reflect on in the future to see how far you have come. It's a fabulous way of measuring your success without relying on misleading indicators like weight or BMI (the body mass index, an over-simplified calculation created by a bloke in the 1800s that's as flawed as a hand-drawn ruler).

The more you tune into your body and what your hormones are telling you during this process, the better. Make a note in your journal, numbering the severity 0 to 9 for each feeling and symptom. This is what you're going to look back on in a few weeks, then a few months and then, potentially, a year from now. This is going to be your reference point, because your success arises from the self – not a number on a scale.

Your journey is unique to you – don't compare it to anyone else's. This is the danger zone in diet culture and social media. If your intuition tells you that you are feeling happier and healthier, you're on the right path.

Now that you have tuned in with how you are feeling, let's explore what can open the doors to optimal health, improved energy, better sleep, and boosted happiness: your hormones. They are your superpower.

Using a notebook or a Notes app on your phone, rate each of the following on a scale from 1–10:

HAPPINESS

Is it easy for you to laugh and smile, or do you feel low, deflated and unhappy?

| 1 | 2 | 3 | 4 | 5 | 6 | 7 | 8 | 9 | 10 |

EXTREMELY UNHAPPY   VERY HAPPY

MOODINESS

Are you experiencing moods swings? Are you easily agitated,
or do you currently feel stable and calm?

| 1 | 2 | 3 | 4 | 5 | 6 | 7 | 8 | 9 | 10 |

EXTREMELY MOODY   VERY STABLE

ENERGY

Do you have sustained energy throughout the day,
or do you often feel tired and sluggish?

| 1 | 2 | 3 | 4 | 5 | 6 | 7 | 8 | 9 | 10 |

FREQUENTLY TIRED   VERY ENERGIZED

BLOATING

Do you currently feel bloated and physically uncomfortable?

| 1 | 2 | 3 | 4 | 5 | 6 | 7 | 8 | 9 | 10 |

EXTREMELY BLOATED   NOT BLOATED AT ALL

CONFIDENCE

Do you feel sure of yourself and your abilities in this moment,
or do you lack confidence and feel uncomfortable in your skin?

| 1 | 2 | 3 | 4 | 5 | 6 | 7 | 8 | 9 | 10 |

VERY SELF-CONSCIOUS   VERY CONFIDENT

BRAIN FOG

Are you having trouble concentrating? Are you losing your train of thought,
or can you easily focus?

| 1 | 2 | 3 | 4 | 5 | 6 | 7 | 8 | 9 | 10 |

INTENSE BRAIN FOG   VERY FOCUSED

SWEET CRAVINGS

Have you been craving sugary foods, particularly a few hours after eating?
Do you find yourself regularly eating sugary foods due to cravings?

| 1 | 2 | 3 | 4 | 5 | 6 | 7 | 8 | 9 | 10 |

EXTREME CRAVINGS   NEUTRAL APPETITE

GET UP AND GO

*Are you eager to hop out of bed in the morning and seize the day, or
do you regularly hit the snooze button?*

1	2	3	4	5	6	7	8	9	10

DIFFICULTY WAKING UP   EASILY WAKE UP

ABILITY TO FALL ASLEEP

*Have you been finding it a challenge to fall asleep,
or are you able to hit your pillow and drift off easily?*

1	2	3	4	5	6	7	8	9	10

DIFFICULTY FALLING ASLEEP   EASILY FALL ASLEEP

STRESS

*Do you feel particularly irritable, angry, tearful, and anxious,
or are you feeling peaceful and calm?*

1	2	3	4	5	6	7	8	9	10

EXTREMELY STRESSED   VERY CALM

SKIN

*Do you currently have clear, healthy-looking skin,
or are you experiencing any breakouts or unusually oily skin?*

1	2	3	4	5	6	7	8	9	10

PROBLEM SKIN   VERY CLEAR SKIN

POSITIVITY

*Does your glass feel half full or half empty? Do you feel grateful and hopeful,
or are you finding it hard to see the positives?*

1	2	3	4	5	6	7	8	9	10

FEELING NEGATIVE   FEELING POSITIVE

PRODUCTIVITY

*Are you able to work efficiently, complete tasks, and work through to-do lists,
or are you finding it hard to get things done?*

1	2	3	4	5	6	7	8	9	10

EXTREMELY UNPRODUCTIVE   EXCEPTIONALLY PRODUCTIVE

RELATIONSHIP WITH FOOD

*Do you feel in control and content about what you're eating, or do you
find yourself overthinking food and associating it with feelings of guilt and shame?*

1	2	3	4	5	6	7	8	9	10

POOR RELATIONSHIP   POSITIVE RELATIONSHIP

Hormones Are
Your Superpower

What are hormones, what do they do, and why are they so powerful?

Your hormones are messengers. More specifically, they are chemical messengers that travel around the body, regulating your physiology and behaviour. Hormones are highly complicated and defining them can be tricky, as some molecules have multiple roles in the body. Vitamin D, for instance, is both a vitamin and a hormone, while serotonin is both a hormone and a neurotransmitter.

No matter how frustrating your symptoms may be, try not to blame your hormones. That is, do not shoot the messenger. I understand how tempting this can be. For years, I blamed my hormones instead of looking at what was causing them to go off balance. Use this opportunity to shift your perspective, and reframe your hormones in a positive light – and we all know the power of good lighting.

The method you will learn is founded on working with your hormones. All healthy relationships begin with understanding, so let's dive in.

CHOLESTEROL: THE HORMONE BUILDER

In the beginning, there was... cholesterol. Think of this as the intro track to your sex hormones; without cholesterol, your sex and steroid hormones would not exist. We call cholesterol the main substrate for sex and steroid hormone biosynthesis – a fancy way of saying that it is the raw material for your steroid hormones. Hormones such as oestrogen, progesterone, testosterone, and cortisol are all derived from the same starting point: cholesterol.

About 80 per cent of your cholesterol is produced by the liver, packaged as lipoproteins – fat and protein parcels – for transport in the bloodstream. The remaining 20 per cent comes from dietary cholesterol in the food you eat.

Cholesterol has many biological functions, carrying out a number of nitty-gritty jobs at a cellular level – synthesizing vitamin D, for one. Every cell in your body has a phospholipid layer (lipid, meaning fat). Cholesterol is needed to maintain optimal cellular membranes by supporting their fluidity and rigidity. Skin disorders (a larger-scale reflection of your membrane) are often a telltale sign that your diet is lacking in essential fats. This is why eating good quality fat and looking after your liver is so integral to hormone health.

HORMONAL PATHWAYS

Next, we meet pregnenolone, which comes from cholesterol. This is the precursor and starting substrate to DHEA, progesterone, cortisol, testosterone, and oestrogen.

This is where we really begin to understand hormones: their creation (known as hormone genesis) and their pathways. There are many steps each hormone has to take before it can set off to deliver its message. When a hormone travels through your body, it heads directly to its target cell and delivers its message via its receptor. It then swiftly exits via the process of detoxification.

HORMONE MAKEUP

Steroid hormones are fat-based hormones derived from cholesterol, including sex hormones (mainly from ovaries) and stress hormones (mainly from adrenals). While adrenal glands can produce some sex hormones, the ovaries sometimes produce adrenal steroids. Sex hormones regulate sexual traits, development and reproduction, while stress hormones control stress response, metabolism, inflammation, and immunity.

Not all hormones are made from fat, though – some come from proteins called **amino acids**. For example, melatonin is an amine hormone derived from tryptophan. Peptide hormones, which are shorter chains of amino acids, help regulate energy balance and metabolism.

THE HORMONE CHAIN

The pathway below shows the basic steps in how steroid hormones are made. This is a simplified version, though – the actual process is much more complex.

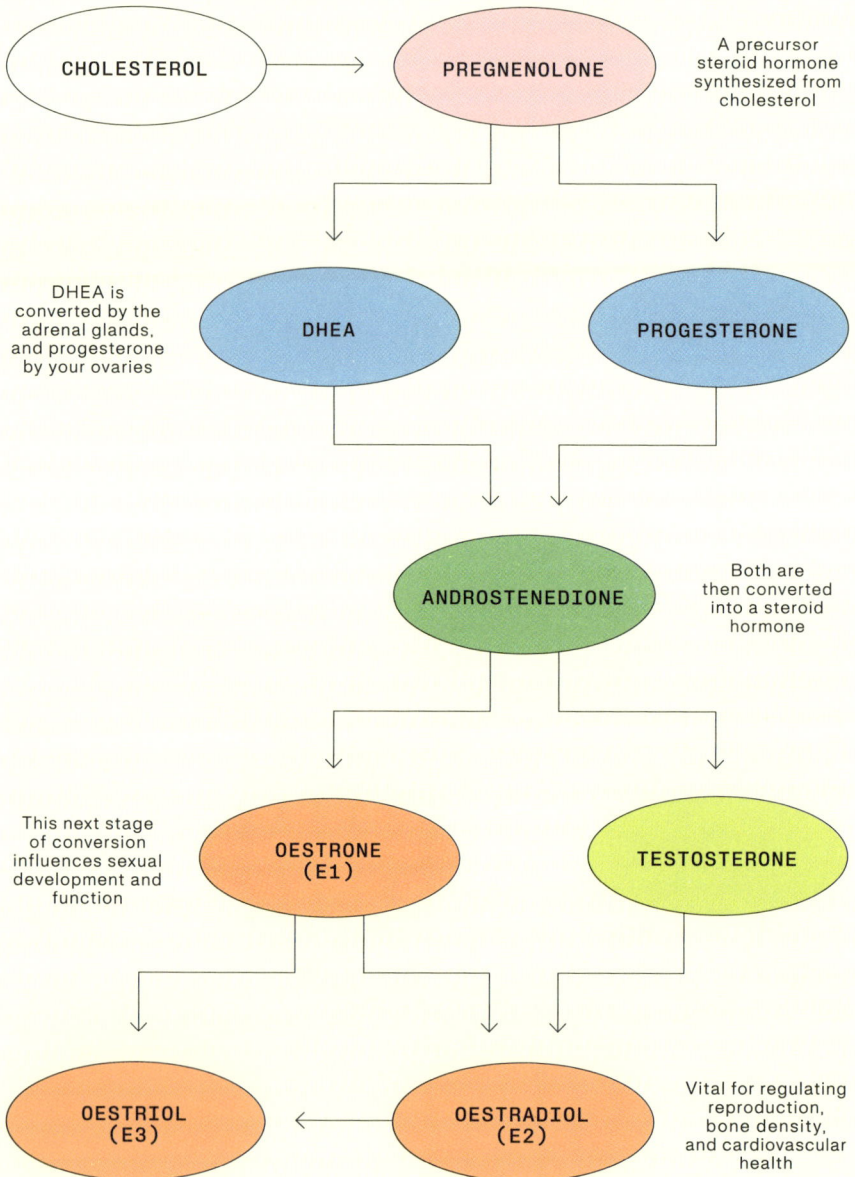

CHOLESTEROL → PREGNENOLONE

A precursor steroid hormone synthesized from cholesterol

DHEA is converted by the adrenal glands, and progesterone by your ovaries

DHEA

PROGESTERONE

ANDROSTENEDIONE

Both are then converted into a steroid hormone

This next stage of conversion influences sexual development and function

OESTRONE (E1)

TESTOSTERONE

OESTRIOL (E3) ← OESTRADIOL (E2)

Vital for regulating reproduction, bone density, and cardiovascular health

For each hormone, there are multiple glands, pathways, enzymes, and catalysts. Even for the same hormone – for instance, progesterone – the journey can vary. Progesterone can be produced in the ovaries after ovulation, for instance, but it can also be formed in the adrenal glands during times of stress.

So, although pregnenolone is the starter hormone to all of your sex hormones, there is no one single pool of pregnenolone that all of your sex and steroid hormones are derived from – it's a web of pathways more complicated than an international airport.

Oestrogen

Oestrogens (estrogens) are sex steroid hormones associated with your female reproductive organs. Made predominantly in your ovaries, they are responsible for developing secondary female sexual characteristics that appear during puberty and sexual maturity. They are also responsible for managing your menstrual cycle – among many other things. From puberty to your reproductive years, perimenopause and beyond, oestrogen influences every key hormonal life stage.

PUBERTY
is the stage at which a child matures into an adult, marked by physical changes like the development of secondary sexual characteristics including breast development, hip widening, and pubic hair growth. It also marks the start of menstruation.

PERIMENOPAUSE
is the transitional phase before menopause, when ovaries gradually become less active. There can be a roller coaster of hormonal changes as sex hormones start to decline, with symptoms such as irregular periods, hot flushes (hot flashes), and mood changes.

MENOPAUSE
is the natural life transition marking the end of a woman's reproductive years, characterized by the cessation of menstruation.

Puberty typically begins between the ages of 8 and 13 in females (this range has seen a change, see p.17). Things then stay pretty steady as your hormones follow their monthly ritual of peaks and troughs (see p.48) up until you experience the midlife metabolic transition of menopause.

Fast-forward a few decades, and you'll see a natural decrease in your sex hormones attributed to perimenopause. This can start as early as your thirties, but typically begins in your late forties.

UNDERSTANDING OESTROGEN

Although we refer to oestrogen as one of your female sex hormones, think about it more as a "life" hormone – this beautiful hormone really looks after you. It's involved with so much more than just your menstrual cycle – it supports your metabolic function, cardiovascular system, neurological system, nervous system, skeletal system, skin health, and energy homeostasis, functioning via a network of oestrogen receptors all over your body.

While we sometimes refer to oestrogen in the singular, there are four types of oestrogen: oestradiol, oestrone, oestriol, and oestetrol. Oestradiol is vital for reproduction and overall health, while oestrone becomes dominant after menopause. Oestriol is mainly produced during pregnancy and oestetrol is produced by the foetal liver during pregnancy.

OESTRADIOL

This is your most abundant form of oestrogen, and the one that starts to drop off as we approach perimenopause. It's sometimes referred to as E2. It's synthesized in the developing follicles of your ovaries after the aromatization of testosterone into oestradiol. This sounds like a mouthful, but in essence, it is created from an androgen. Oestradiol peaks during ovulation in your follicular phase, helping your uterine lining to thicken. It then drops during your period, and again during menopause.

Aromatisation is a fancy word for describing the conversion of an androgen hormone to an oestrogen. It's the fundamental pathway for the synthesis of oestradiol. An enzyme called aromatase is produced in response

ANDROGENS

"Androgens" is the collective term for the group of male sexual characteristic hormones, like a herd of sheep or a flamboyance of flamingos. The term "androgen" refers to any steroid hormone that has masculinizing effects.

to FSH (follicle-stimulating hormone), and this enzyme then converts androgens produced by the the cells to oestradiol. Think of it as a total transformation. This is the main way that your body creates oestrogen.

OESTRONE

This is the last oestrogen standing in terms of your hormone lifecycle, as its production continues after menopause. It's referred to as E1. Your ovaries produce it in small amounts, but it is mainly formed via a conversion from androgens.

OESTRIOL & OESTETROL

These are your pregnancy-only oestrogen hormones. Oestriol is made from a male hormone called DHEA-S, which is actually derived from your unborn child's DHEA-S androgens. It is also made from dietary cholesterol, which is converted to pregnenolone and progesterone in the placenta Oestriol is created from the foetal adrenal glands, while oestetrol is made by the foetal liver. Both are then circulated into mummy's circulation through the placenta. Pretty cool!

Oestradiol is 80 times as potent as oestriol, and 12 times as potent as oestrone.

All of the above can contribute to oestrogen dominance, but typically oestrogen dominance is driven by poor detoxification. This is why you are going to be learning to love your liver!

THE MANY ROLES OF OESTROGEN

Oestrogen acts on multiple systems, from your fatty tissue to your brain, your bones, skeletal muscle, liver, and your immune cells, regulating essential functions throughout your body.

Both puberty and perimenopause are periods of major transition, triggered by shifts in oestrogen production. Though separated by decades, each represents a significant developmental transition with neurological as well as reproductive impacts. And for the lucky ones with daughters at home, you may even experience these two female hormonal shifts happening under the same roof at the same time!

A recent study looking into this link drew a fascinating parallel with these two natural shifts, concluding that the transition state of perimenopause is similar to the developing neurological dysfunction exhibited at puberty. This demonstrates the fundamental role played by oestrogen in your overall wellbeing, as significant hormonal shifts can increase vulnerability to anxiety, depression, and psychiatric disorders. This highlights the deep-rooted link between oestrogen and your neurological system.

The higher levels of oestrogen in women are thought to contribute to longer lifespans when compared to men. Oestrogen also has a big role to play with the intake of food through its relationship with leptin, a hormone that signals fullness. It also influences your fat distribution and energy expenditure, closely linking this hormone with your weight and body shape.

OESTROGEN IMBALANCE

Oestrogen is associated with many bodily processes. An imbalance can therefore lead to a vicious cycle in which one oestrogen-reliant mechanism can play into another and create a bubbling pot of worsening symptoms. Conversely, the good news is that when one area starts to thrive, so does another, leading to greater overall harmony.

Oestrogen is secreted at differing rates depending on where you are in your cycle, as well as where you may be in your lifespan (e.g. closer to puberty or perimenopause) or where you are in relation to other significant life events (e.g. pregnancy and the postnatal phase).

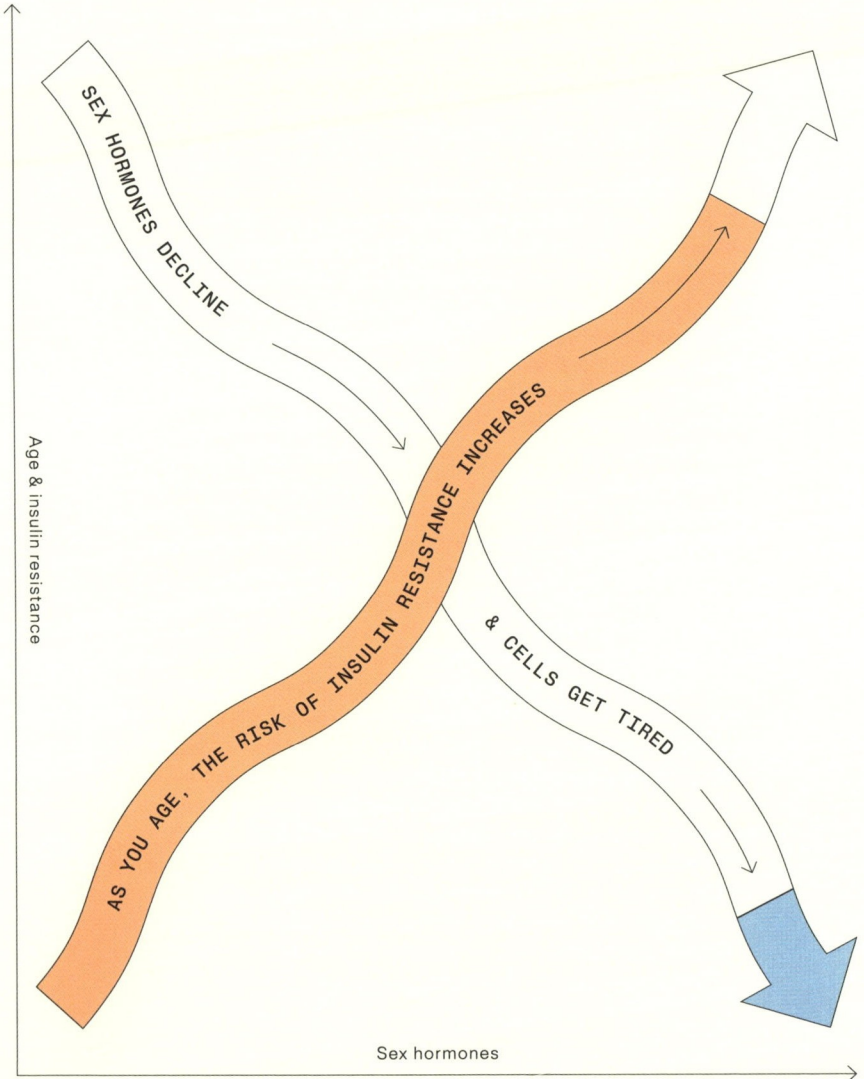

**INSULIN RESISTANCE
VS SEX HORMONE REDUCTION**
As you age and your oestrogen
levels drop, your risk of insulin
resistance increases. It's
essential to acknowledge this
risk, and counteract it with the
right diet and lifestyle choices
(see chapter 3, p.116).

Age & insulin resistance

SEX HORMONES DECLINE

AS YOU AGE, THE RISK OF INSULIN RESISTANCE INCREASES

& CELLS GET TIRED

Sex hormones

As mentioned in our discussion of PCOS (see pp.6–8), this is why one must exercise particular caution around metabolic syndrome, primarily insulin resistance, during certain phases of your hormone lifespan. This is especially true if you have PCOS, hypothyroidism, or if you are postmenopausal, as there is an increased risk of developing metabolic syndrome.

Metabolic syndrome is a collective term for health issues that put you at greater risk of type 2 diabetes or conditions that affect your heart or blood vessels. These include insulin resistance, cardiovascular disease, high blood pressure, and non-alcoholic fatty liver disease.

OESTROGEN DEFICIENCY

The less oestrogen being produced by your body, the more at risk you are of metabolic syndrome. Research has demonstrated that oestradiol improves insulin sensitivity, which is why women are at greater risk of developing insulin resistance during the perimenopause and in other conditions involving low oestrogen.

To put it simply – the less oestrogen in your system, the quicker you will age.

The risk of metabolic syndrome is also true for trans people who have undergone gender-affirming hormone (GAHT) therapy to improve their quality of life and reduce gender dysphoria. A fascinating 2024 study explored whether oestradiol and testosterone are associated with the development of metabolic syndrome in transgender veterans compared with cisgender veterans. What was concluded is that transmasculine individuals (who would have reduced oestrogen levels due to testosterone hormone therapy) had a higher risk of metabolic syndrome compared to transfeminine individuals (who would have increased oestrogen levels due to hormone therapy). So trans women, having higher levels of oestrogen, had the lowest risk of metabolic syndrome. Here, the power of oestrogen strikes again: higher oestradiol was associated with a reduced metabolic syndrome risk, whereas lower oestradiol was associated with increased risk.

This study showcases why insulin resistance plays such a pivotal role in your hormonal health as well as general health, and how your stage in the hormone lifespan plays a crucial role in determining your risk of insulin resistance.

WHEN ARE YOU MOST LIKELY TO EXPERIENCE LOW OESTROGEN?*

Oestrogen levels can fall naturally during the menstrual cycle or decline as you age, but can also be a symptom of conditions like PCOS.

Postnatal phase and while breastfeeding

Perimenopause

Menopause and postmenopause

Thyroid dysfunction

Polycystic ovarian syndrome (PCOS)

Taking the oral contraceptive pill

Experiencing a highly stressful life event

Hysterectomy

Low levels of the aromatase enzyme (which converts testosterone into oestrogen)

Nutrient deficiencies, particularly vitamin D

WHAT DOES OESTROGEN DEFICIENCY LOOK LIKE?*

Oestrogen deficiency is a mediator of poor health and metabolic syndrome, which leaves individuals predisposed to obesity, type 2 diabetes, and certain cancers including breast and colon.

Hot flushes

Irregular periods

Difficulty sleeping

Night sweats

Palpitations

Depression

Anxiety

Changed body shape

Weight gain

Skin changes, including dry and itchy skin

Recurrent thrush (yeast infections)

Muscle aches and joint pain

Bacterial vaginosis

Low libido

Recurrent UTIs (urinary tract infections)

Vaginal dryness and pain, itching or discomfort during sex

Headaches and migraines

The list goes on...

* symptoms include, but are not limited to, this list

CAN WE HAVE TOO MUCH OESTROGEN?

You might now be thinking that the answer to all our problems is to overload ourselves with this seeming elixir of youth called oestrogen. It doesn't work like that, though. At the other end of the spectrum, it is completely possible to have excess levels of oestrogen in the body. This usually happensif oestrogen is not being properly metabolized and eliminated by your liver, gut, and your bowel movements.

Below are a few other factors that can influence excess oestrogen:

Adrenal dysfunction

Excessively high levels of the aromatase enzyme (which converts testosterone into oestrogen)

Gut dysbiosis

High exposure to plastics, products, pesticides, microplastics, and tap water containing environmental oestrogens and xenoestrogens

High percentage of body fat

Insulin resistance

Ovarian tumours

Suboptimal detoxification

Oestrogen dominance theory refers to normal or high levels of oestrogen with little to no counterbalancing progesterone. While not a conventional medical term, an imbalanced oestrogen-to-progesterone ratio can lead to hormone-related symptoms. Inadequate ovulation can result in low progesterone, allowing oestrogen to dominate. Even with low overall oestrogen, a skewed ratio can still cause symptoms.

ELEVATED OESTROGEN, HISTAMINE, AND ALLERGIES

Oestrogen has a significant influence on your immune function – this can include skewing your immune response toward allergies. One example of this is the production of histamine. Histamine is a chemical that mediates your allergy response. It is released from the immune system during allergic reactions, causing symptoms such as rashes, itching, runny nose, and sneezing. Oestrogen stimulates the release of histamine, and also inhibits the enzyme diamine oxidase (DAO), which breaks down histamine in the gut.

WHAT DOES EXCESS OESTROGEN LOOK LIKE?*

PMS	Sleep disturbances
Endometriosis (a pro-inflammatory condition that is highly oestrogen-dependent)	Bloating
	Weight gain
	Breast tenderness
Heavy periods	Breast cysts
Irritability and mood swings	Fibroids
Headaches and migraines	Thyroid disorders
Low libido	A risk of oestrogen-driven cancers

Environmental oestrogens such as xenoestrogens, found in plastics, may increase histamine and contribute to the development of atopic disorders like asthma, while certain foods high in histamine – including alcohol, fermented foods, canned foods, and smoked foods – can also exacerbate symptoms.

Histamine intolerance occurs when the body has trouble breaking down histamine, which then leads to further build-up in the body. This can manifest as a number of symptoms (see right). I see a large number of clients in my clinic who struggle with histamine intolerance alongside endometriosis and ovarian cysts, as well as during perimenopause.

* symptoms include, but are not limited to, this list

WHAT DOES HISTAMINE INTOLERANCE LOOK LIKE?

Itchy skin, rashes, hives

Urticaria (a common skin condition appearing as itchy wheals on the skin)

Diarrhoea (diarrhea)

Bloating

Nausea or vomiting

Headaches

Runny or stuffy nose

Shortness of breath

Fatigue

Progesterone

Progesterone is the other major player among your sex hormones and cycle. It works in tandem with oestrogen to support a healthy menstrual cycle, as well as your immune function and supporting pregnancy –its presenceis a prerequisite for embryo implantation and a healthy pregnancy.

Progesterone stays relatively low just before ovulation, and then peaks after ovulation during your luteal phase. This rise is in response to the surge of luteinizing hormone (which triggers the release of an egg) as oestrogen levels start to drop off.

Just after ovulation, something called your corpus luteum appears, which is a collection of cells that form around your ovaries each month. Progesterone is mainly produced by the corpus luteum, a temporary endocrine gland that prepares the uterus for pregnancy. If fertilization doesn't occur, it disappears after a few days. Progesterone can also be made by the adrenal cortex and, during pregnancy, by the placenta.

PROGESTERONE AND PREGNANCY

Progesterone has a few jobs, but its main task is to support and maintain a pregnancy, if one occurs. It does this by creating a healthy uterine lining to sustain embryo implantation and support the pregnancy. A lack of progesterone can also sadly lead to pregnancy loss. If you ovulate and then do not fall pregnant, you then see the downward spiral of this hormone ahead of your period. This drop in progesterone can be a factor in premenstrual syndrome (PMS), which can present as bloating and feeling irritable.

SIGNS OF PROGESTERONE DEFICIENCY

Low levels of progesterone can be linked to bloating, as progesterone exerts an inhibitory role on the gut by slowing it down, in part by elevating nitric oxide synthesis. This is why the frequency of your bowel movements is majorly slowed by pregnancy, when progesterone levels soar – it can also be a common symptom of PMS.

PREMENSTRUAL DYSPHORIC DISORDER (PMDD)

PMDD is the most severe form of PMS, but the two should not be confused. A distinct, life-disrupting mood disorder, PMDD shares some symptoms with PMS but operates in a different stratosphere. It involves heightened sensitivity to normal hormonal shifts during the menstrual cycle. It is linked to fluctuations in progesterone, allopregnanolone (a progesterone metabolite), oestrogen, testosterone and neurotransmitters like serotonin, GABA, and glutamate.

Symptoms affecting mood, behaviour, and the physical body typically intensify six days before a period and peak two days before bleeding, though timings can vary.

Like many other hormones, progesterone has a protective role – remember how we said hormones have got your back? It plays a part in reducing your risk of ovarian cancer, and it works in tandem with vitamin D for sequential and effective regulation of your immune system.

PROGESTERONE AND THE BRAIN

With big links to your GABA receptors, progesterone is often referred to as your "chill out" hormone. GABA is a wonderful neurotransmitter that can produce a calming effect by blocking certain signals in your central nervous system and slowing down your brain. Think of it like taking a deep, calming breath, or being wrapped up in a warm hug. Alcohol acts on this same transmitter, hence that warm fuzzy calm feeling that accompanies a glass of bubbly.

Progesterone – and one of its metabolites called allopregnanolone – directly interacts with your GABA receptors and can induce sedative, anti-depressant effects.

PROGESTERONE AND MENTAL HEALTH

Your brain cells also have progesterone receptors, which contribute to managing your emotions. So, if there are low levels of progesterone, there will also be low levels of its metabolites – this naturally starts to happen in perimenopause or if you are ovulating regularly. And here we have one of the major links between mood and progesterone: low levels of progesterone play an essential part in feelings of anxiety, inducing mood disorders like premenstrual syndrome (PMS) and premenstrual dysphoric disorder (PMDD).

This is why women are particularly vulnerable to mental health challenges after giving birth and during perimenopause and beyond – both cases involve a natural drop in progesterone. Taking away your previously abundant sex hormones can be an emotional shock to the system.

Postpartum depression is connected to the sudden drop in steroid hormones; once the placenta and baby are delivered, the abundant flow of progesterone and oestrogen goes with them.

In an incredible recent development, allopregnanolone has been approved as a medication for postpartum depression in the US by the Food and Drug Administration (FDA). As we said earlier, this is the spin-off hormone that has the best links to GABA, which plays a key role in regulating mood. It has shown great results when compared to medicated hormone replacement therapy with progestins (medicated progesterone) – this type of synthetic progesterone won't be able to create a spin-off allopregnalone. So, unlike your natural progesterone, progestins cannot be metabolized by the body as allopregnanolone, which means that you miss out on all the mood-boosting derivatives that come with your body's own hormone.

Natural progesterone has also been linked to progestins' unfavourable impacts on mood, which of course is quite the opposite of the intended effect. Progesterone and its sidekick metabolites play an important role in mood fluctuations in women, but more conversations and more research into this relationship is needed to provide better medical solutions for women alongside the nutrition and lifestyle changes that we already know to be effective.

WHAT CAN LOW PROGESTERONE LOOK LIKE?*

Anxiety	Bloating
Low mood	Hot flushes
Irregular cycles	Disrupted sleep
Miscarriage	Irritability and mood swings
Headaches and migraines	Spotting and brown blood present at the start of a period
Infertility	

UNDERSTANDING WHY YOUR PROGESTERONE MIGHT BE LOW

So, why might your progesterone be low? Let's look at the main creation point: ovulation. If you're not ovulating regularly or at all, you won't be producing a corpus luteum – the source of your progesterone, impacting how much or how little of the hormone you produce. A new corpus luteum forms each time you ovulate. This is why the best way to increase your progesterone is to boost ovulation through optimal oestrogen.

If you have low levels of progesterone relative to oestrogen, this can increase the risk of oestrogen becoming dominant – which is when things can become problematic. This imbalance disrupts the complex regulatory mechanisms of the two hormones, and can even cause progesterone resistance in the body. Oestrogen and progesterone work in harmony to regulate your reproductive system, especially in maintaining your uterine lining, also known as your endometrium. During every cycle of your reproductive years, your uterine lining undergoes a pretty astonishing makeover.

*symptoms include, but are not limited to, this list

PROGESTERONE AND THE MENSTRUAL CYCLE

The female reproductive system is amazing: a lifetime of dynamic remodelling is spent regenerating, proliferating, and shedding. This process is driven by the ultimate tag team, oestrogen and progesterone. Oestrogen promotes the repair and proliferation, or growth, of your uterine lining or endometrium. After ovulation, progesterone steps up to thicken your uterine lining. As progesterone levels continue to rise in the hope that you may become pregnant, so too does its ratio to oestrogen.

A common issue with this duo is that oestrogen can overshadow progesterone. If oestrogen is dominant, we can become less sensitive to progesterone, which can compromise fertility and drive gynaecological conditions like endometriosis.

The relationship between oestrogen and progesterone is vital (see p.45), and one that we want to support.

Look after your cortisol and your insulin, which will then help you nurture your testosterone and in turn support your oestrogen. This will support your ovulation and your relationship with progesterone – it's a team effort!

The Female Reproductive System

Before we move on to learn about the other key hormones, let's look at one of the primary roles of oestrogen and progesterone: regulating the menstrual cycle.

We women are rhythmical creatures. This is going to become even more apparent in Pillar Five on p.184, when we learn how to support your circadian rhythm. As we've just become acquainted with oestrogen and progesterone, let's look at what happens to your body over the course of your life.

When puberty hits, often between the ages of 8 and 14, the child's body matures into that of an adult, a process accompanied by hormonal surges and physical change.

MENSTRUATION

This is the first phase of your cycle. This is where you shed the lining of the uterus if pregnancy has not occurred. Oestrogen and progesterone levels at this stage are low, and you may be experiencing cramps, tender breasts, mood swings, headaches, and fatigue – all those classic PMS symptoms that can be exacerbated by things like diet-induced inflammation, or conditions like endometriosis and PCOS.

FOLLICULAR PHASE

You then enter into your follicular phase, beginning on the first day of your period, where follicles mature in the ovaries and oestrogen levels rise to prepare the uterine lining for potential pregnancy. Your hypothalamus signals your pituitary gland to release follicle-stimulating hormone (FSH). This hormone prompts your ovaries to produce a batch of small follicles, but only the most advanced egg will mature, while the rest will be reabsorbed by your body. This process is triggered by a surge in oestradiol, which thickens your uterine lining – the perfect environment for an embryo to grow. As ovulation nears, your libido may also start to increase. Time for an "everything" shower...

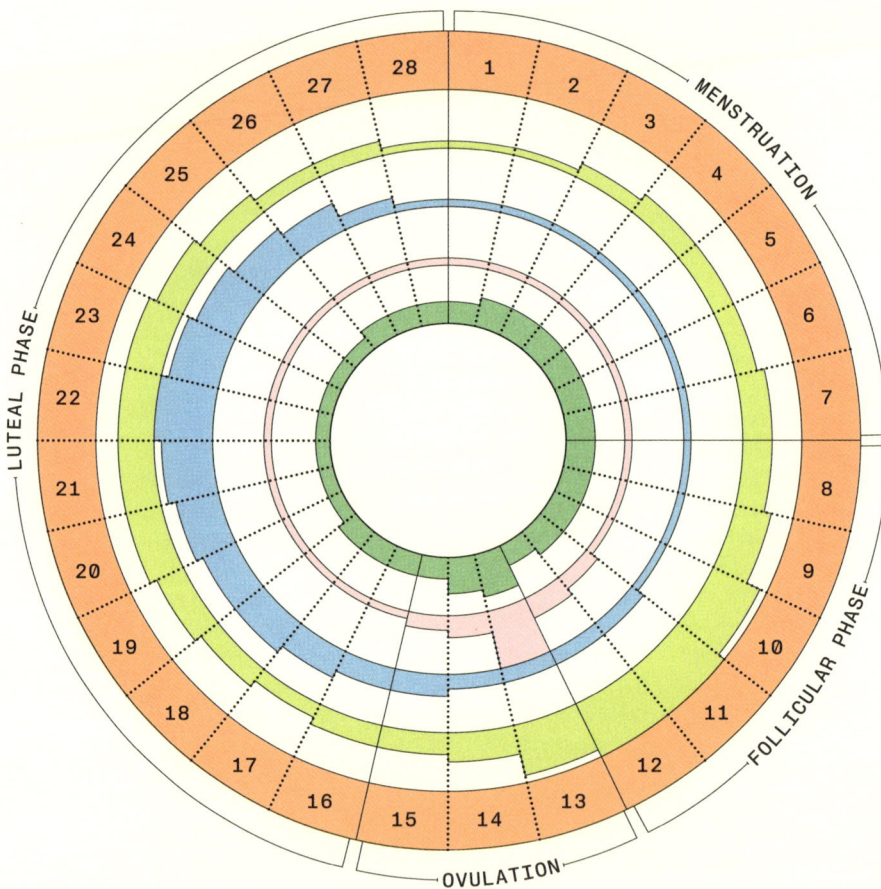

THE MENSTRUAL CYCLE
This diagram shows a "typical" menstrual cycle, but in reality it can vary widely. Ovulation, for instance, usually begins on day 14, but in clinic, I see anything from day 10 to day 19.

MENSTRUATION

FOLLICULAR PHASE

OVULATION

LUTEAL PHASE

Oestrogen levels

Progesterone levels

LH levels

FSH levels

OVULATION

All the rising oestradiol then triggers your pituitary gland to secrete luteinizing hormone (LH). This is what starts the process of ovulation, and the mature egg makes its journey down the fallopian tube with the aim of being fertilized by sperm. During ovulation there's a slight rise in basal body temperature, and sometimes thicker, sticky vaginal discharge that may help give swimming sperm more of a fighting chance. Research has indicated that women have also been found to report greater sexual attraction to men with masculine features when near ovulation relative to the luteal phase. This shift is believed to stem from evolutionary biology and is linked to the reproductive instinct. Studies measuring scent attractiveness have also found that female scents change throughout our cycle. Research shows that, on average, women's scents are perceived as more attractive around the time of ovulation, compared to other days in their cycle. There is also a positive correlation between higher levels of oestradiol and the attractiveness of these scents, suggesting that hormone fluctuations may come with sexy scent cues.

But what about your own sense of smell? This tends to peak during ovulation. This heightened sense of smell during your peak fertility window is meant to draw you to the male pheromone androsterone. Fun fact: one of the signs that ovulation is imminent is a heightened sense of smell. It can even put you off your own perfume!

LUTEAL PHASE

After ovulation, the luteal phase begins with the egg travelling down the fallopian tube toward the uterus to be fertilized by sperm. It's at this point that the follicle changes. The empty sac closes off, turns yellow, and transforms into a new structure called the corpus luteum. The corpus luteum releases progesterone and oestrogen. This is why women with conditions like PCOS can have low levels of progesterone – if you are not ovulating, you miss out on this stage where progesterone is produced. The body is prepped for a potential pregnancy by progesterone, which, as we know, can have a calming effect through its links to GABA.

After ovulation, progesterone is the dominant hormone. At this stage your body may give you clues if your progesterone levels are low. If this is the case, you may notice spotting before your period, irregular cycles, heavier or longer periods, or even short cycles due to a short luteal phase.

If pregnancy does not occur, the corpus luteum will shrink away and be resorbed. This then will trigger a drop in oestrogen and progesterone, which causes the onset of your period. The uterine lining will then be shed.

PMS AND PERIOD PAIN

While you are menstruating, you may feel more emotional – just one of those classic PMS symptoms. There is even an associated higher risk of mood disorders via oestrogen-serotonin regulation.

Clinical trials have shown that serotonin precursors significantly increase between days 7 to 11, and days 17 to 19 of the menstrual cycle – another shout-out to why PMS is closely linked to mood.

WHAT DOES PMS LOOK LIKE?*

Bloating	Headaches
Breast tenderness or changes in breasts	Low libido
Changes in skin, like acne or dryness	Mood swings, sadness, or anxiety

If period pain is an issue for you, there is a chance that it is linked to the change in your oestrogen and progesterone levels before a period. The imbalance of these two hormones impact the entire bodily system, including brain neurotransmitters (principally serotonin and GABA). Pain is of course complex and subjective, but low levels of serotonin can be linked to pain and pain disorders.

Low progesterone can potentially impact your emotional and physical wellbeing, which, alongside typical PMS symptoms, can manifest as pain.

*symptoms include, but are not limited to, this list

Many of us experience period pain, but it can present in different ways, from womb (uterine) contractions to inflammation, or a heightened sensitivity to pain caused by hormonal changes. First, identify what is causing your pain. Is it period pain, back pain or something more complex? It is important to first rule out any potential underlying issues such as endometriosis, fibroids, and pelvic inflammatory disease.

Period pain can occur when your womb wall starts to contract with more intensity to promote the shedding of your womb lining. As this happens, the flow of oxygen to your womb can be affected. Without oxygen, the tissues in your womb release chemicals that trigger pain, and also a group of inflammatory lipids called prostaglandins.

These lipids encourage your womb muscles to contract even more, further increasing the level of pain. The more prostaglandins produced, the more inflammation and pain. It's unclear exactly why some women produce more prostaglandins than others – it's likely a combination of genetics, the cyclic hormone drop and additional lifestyle factors such as smoking, poor diet, and alcohol.

CAUSES OF PERIOD PAIN

When it comes to pain, the key factor is inflammation. We're going to dive into inflammation a little later in this chapter (see p.56), but it's worth saying now that reducing inflammation in your body takes time. A sudden bought of period pain won't be tamed by one anti-inflammatory turmeric latte. If your pain interferes with your life, communicate this to your doctor and stick to your guns – if you get brushed off, seek a second opinion. Once you have ruled out any serious conditions via your doctor, shift your diet and lifestyle to embrace one that reduces inflammation. You'll learn how to do this in chapter Three. But remember that patience is crucial.

You can't change your own genetics, but you can influence how they manifest. Endometriosis and period pain may be influenced by genetics, but the environment that you create for your body via diet and lifestyle can still have a positive impact. An unsuitable diet can actually increase prostaglandin production, while an anti-inflammatory diet helps inhibit prostaglandin production.

Testosterone

Welcome to the most abundant sex hormone in your body: testosterone. I'm also a big fan of this one, because testosterone is a precursor to oestrogen, your life hormone. It's got a set of pretty important jobs to do: improving your mood and sex drive, supporting your muscle and bone mass and, with new research highlighting its role in endometrial physiology, helping to maintain, repair, and build your reproductive tissues.

Together with your other androgen hormones, testosterone plays a vital role in the maintenance of your reproductive system and cardiac health. While testosterone aids your body's resilience and power, when it goes rogue (which, we'll see, can happen easily) it can be hard to handle.

TESTOSTERONE HAS SOME IMPORTANT FUNCTIONS, INCLUDING:

Acting as a precursor to oestrogen synthesis

Boosting libido in women

Improving mood and energy

Maintaining bone density and muscle mass

Protecting cognitive function

Like oestrogen, testosterone is produced by the ovaries and adrenal glands. You have androgen (the group of hormones that includes testosterone) receptors all over your body and throughout your brain, and testosterone's effects are wide-ranging.

Testosterone can influence your mental clarity, strengthening nerves in the brain and contributing to cognitive sharpness. It also positively impacts the brain and memory by aiding blood supply and strengthening your arteries. Healthy levels of testosterone are directly linked to higher bone mineral density.

Testosterone is also a key player in your sex drive, maintaining optimal levels of sexual desire. It can even play a role in your sexual gratification. It does this by increasing dopamine levels in the central nervous system and other feel-good neurotransmitters such as serotonin.

Testosterone is transported around the body bound to proteins like sex hormone-binding globulin (SHBG) or albumin, though some exist as unbound "free testosterone", an active hormone easily absorbed by tissues. Elevated free testosterone levels, known as hyperandrogenism, can lead to symptoms like acne, excess facial and body hair, hair thinning or balding, mood swings, and depression. It can also disrupt menstrual cycles, causing irregular periods or anovulation (absence of ovulation).

Testosterone levels generally remain stable throughout the menstrual cycle, with a slight rise around ovulation. During perimenopause, though, reduced ovarian function causes testosterone levels to decline. This drop is further amplified as the body converts more testosterone into oestradiol to compensate for declining oestrogen levels, reflecting testosterone's role as an oestrogen precursor.

I've dealt with out-of-control testosterone production myself during my own journey with PCOS, and I often see it in my private clinic. With an excess of androgens comes a number of symptoms that can negatively impact your quality of life. Many of these symptoms can affect your confidence and quality of life.

WHAT CAN EXCESS TESTOSTERONE LOOK LIKE?

Acne	Irregular or absent periods
Decreased breast size	Male pattern baldness
Decreased or increased libido	Mood swings
Hirsutism (excess hair growth)	Weight gain

Who else on the androgen scene is worth noting? Along with testosterone, meet the rest of the gang: DHT, DHEA, and DHEA-S.

> **ANDROSTENEDIONE**
>
> Androstenedione is part of the androgen family
> as it's a crucial sex-steroid precursor, but it has weak androgenic
> effects on the body. It plays a key role as a precursor in the
> production of both testosterone and oestrogen, helping
> to convert these hormones in the body.

DHT

DHT is the most potent form of androgen. It is considered
to be a pure androgen as, unlike testosterone, it cannot
convert to oestrogen. It's produced from testosterone
through an enzyme called 5-alpha reductase, located
in the peripheral tissues of the body (like your liver) where
it exerts its effects. DHT has approximately double the
binding affinity to androgen receptors – where hormones
deliver their message – which means that its message is
heard louder and prouder. Although DHT is present and
often elevated in many individuals, it actually doesn't seem
to play a significant role in the physiology of women.

DHT does, however, drive a lot of the symptoms listed
above, particularly acne and excess hair growth. In males,
this hormone is the driving force behind sebaceous gland
activity (oily skin), male pattern baldness and hair thinning,
and body, facial, and pubic hair growth. This is why high
levels of this particular hormone can be so frustrating for
women, causing most of the symptoms experienced by men.

DHEA AND DHEA-S

DHEA (dehydroepiandrosterone) and its metabolite, DHEA-S (dehydroepiandrosterone sulphate), are both important hormones in the body. They are both precursor hormones that may be converted into oestrogens or weak androgens – so, both oestrogen and testosterone depend upon it. They are predominately made by your adrenals, and play a role in your insulin sensitivity and muscle mass. Your adrenals are glands that sit just above the kidney, and also produce cortisol. DHEA-S can be elevated for someone with a PCOS profile, or for someone experiencing adrenal dysfunction.

WHAT CAN HIGH LEVELS
OF DHEA-S LOOK LIKE?*

Acne

Irregular and/or missed periods

Hirsutism (excess hair growth)

Male pattern baldness

WHAT CAN LOW LEVELS
OF DHEA-S LOOK LIKE?*

Diabetes

Low libido

Vaginal dryness

WHEN ARE YOU MOST LIKELY TO EXPERIENCE HIGH ANDROGENS?

Adrenal tumours can cause the adrenals to overproduce androgens

Congenital adrenal hyperplasia, a group of genetic conditions affecting the adrenal glands and causing them to produce too much testosterone and other androgen hormones

Ovarian tumours can cause the ovaries to overproduce androgens

Polycystic ovarian syndrome (PCOS)

*symptoms include, but are not limited to, this list

Cortisol

Mighty cortisol, often misunderstood, is produced by your adrenal glands. Cortisol works like an override button; it's loud, it's big and, as it has receptors all over the place, it can affect pretty much every organ in your body, giving you almost superhuman survival power in life-threatening situations. While commonly associated with stress, cortisol influences motivation and is essential for critical bodily functions like managing your sleep-wake cycle and controlling inflammation. However, when cortisol levels are elevated or dysregulated, they can cause health issues instead of resolving them.

The goal isn't to eliminate cortisol from the body – instead, finding balance is key. Alongside insulin, cortisol sits at the top of the hormone regulatory hierarchy. This means that if cortisol or insulin become dysregulated, it can have a major ripple-out effect and your other hormones will follow along.

CORTISOL DAY BY DAY

Cortisol levels naturally fluctuate throughout the day. Ideally, it peaks in the morning to wake you up (this is called your cortisol awakening response), and gradually declines towards the evening, aligning with your body's internal 24-hour clock. This daily rhythm, known as the diurnal rhythm, is regulated by a communication network between your hypothalamus, pituitary, and adrenal glands, known as the HPA (hypothalamic-pituitary-adrenal) axis. It works to maintain balance within the body by regulating your immune function, energy, digestion, and mood, including your sexual drive and emotional health.

Cortisol's messaging can affect your entire body, transmitting signals as loud as a foghorn when elevated. When cortisol levels rise, this can override the body's natural rhythm, alerting your mind and other hormones – especially androgens – in a way that's hard to ignore. One thing's for sure – your body will let you know when cortisol levels are high.

CHRONIC STRESS AND CORTISOL

A potent anti-inflammatory, cortisol is also produced in response to stressful situations as well as in controlling inflammation.

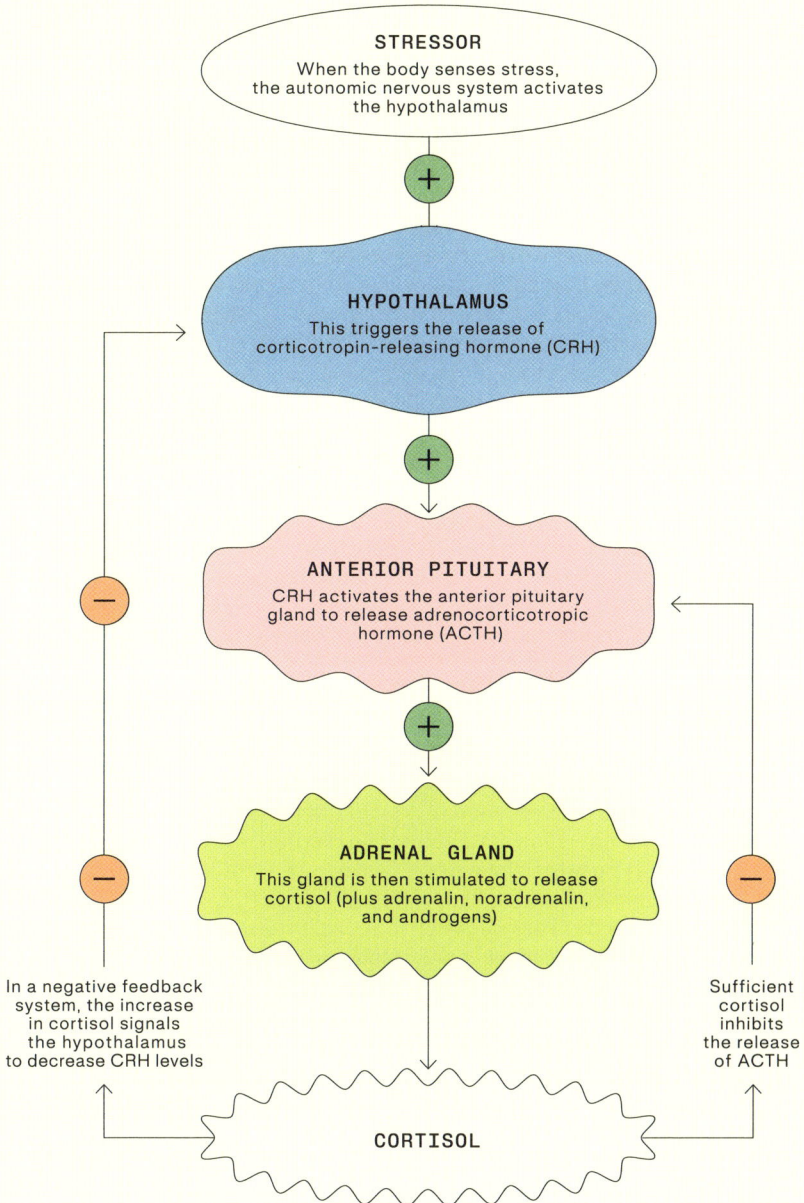

HPA AXIS
The HPA axis is your body's
stress-response system,
connecting your brain and
adrenal glands to regulate
stress hormones such
as cortisol.

(—) Negative feedback

(+) Activation

STRESSOR
When the body senses stress,
the autonomic nervous system activates
the hypothalamus

(+)

HYPOTHALAMUS
This triggers the release of
corticotropin-releasing hormone (CRH)

(+)

ANTERIOR PITUITARY
CRH activates the anterior pituitary
gland to release adrenocorticotropic
hormone (ACTH)

(—)

(+)

ADRENAL GLAND
This gland is then stimulated to release
cortisol (plus adrenalin, noradrenalin,
and androgens)

(—)

(—)

In a negative feedback
system, the increase
in cortisol signals
the hypothalamus
to decrease CRH levels

Sufficient
cortisol
inhibits
the release
of ACTH

CORTISOL

Cortisol aids your stress response, increasing blood sugar when needed, regulating your metabolism and reducing inflammation. When your body feels it is under threat, cortisol is released. Any physical or psychological stimuli that disrupt homeostasis – your body's stable internal environment – results in a stress response.

MODERN STRESS AND CORTISOL

Sources of stress have changed quite a bit over the last few centuries, though. Sabre-tooth tigers have been replaced by deadline-driven office work, global crises, and financial worries. But your body hasn't evolved to handle these new, often psychological stresses; to the body, stress is more black and white, and intense anxiety about any of the above will be classed as a threat.

What happens when your body goes into this state? Once you sense fear, the amygdala in your brain responds by sending a message to your hypothalamus, which activates the autonomic nervous system. In this case, it is your sympathetic nervous system. This triggers the rapid release of cortisol and adrenaline, causing your heart rate to increase, your breathing to speed up, and your liver to release sugar into your bloodstream for an energy boost. Pain perception decreases, your pupils dilate, and your hearing sharpens – you're ready to fight for your life!

CORTISOL AND MENTAL HEALTH

While cortisol is vital during a life-or-death situation, when we are continually stressed over a longer period of time we can experience a constant drip-feed of this hormone, driving disease, inflammation, and endocrine disorders, as well as weight gain, belly fat, and a more rounded, puffy face shape sometimes called "moon face".

Research on severe depression in midlife women during perimenopause found especially elevated cortisol levels in the morning and evening. Deviations from the ideal gentle rise and fall of cortisol – such as consistently high levels of cortisol or a "flatlined" pattern where the hormone remains at one level throughout the day – are associated with depression and anxiety. Evidence shows that women

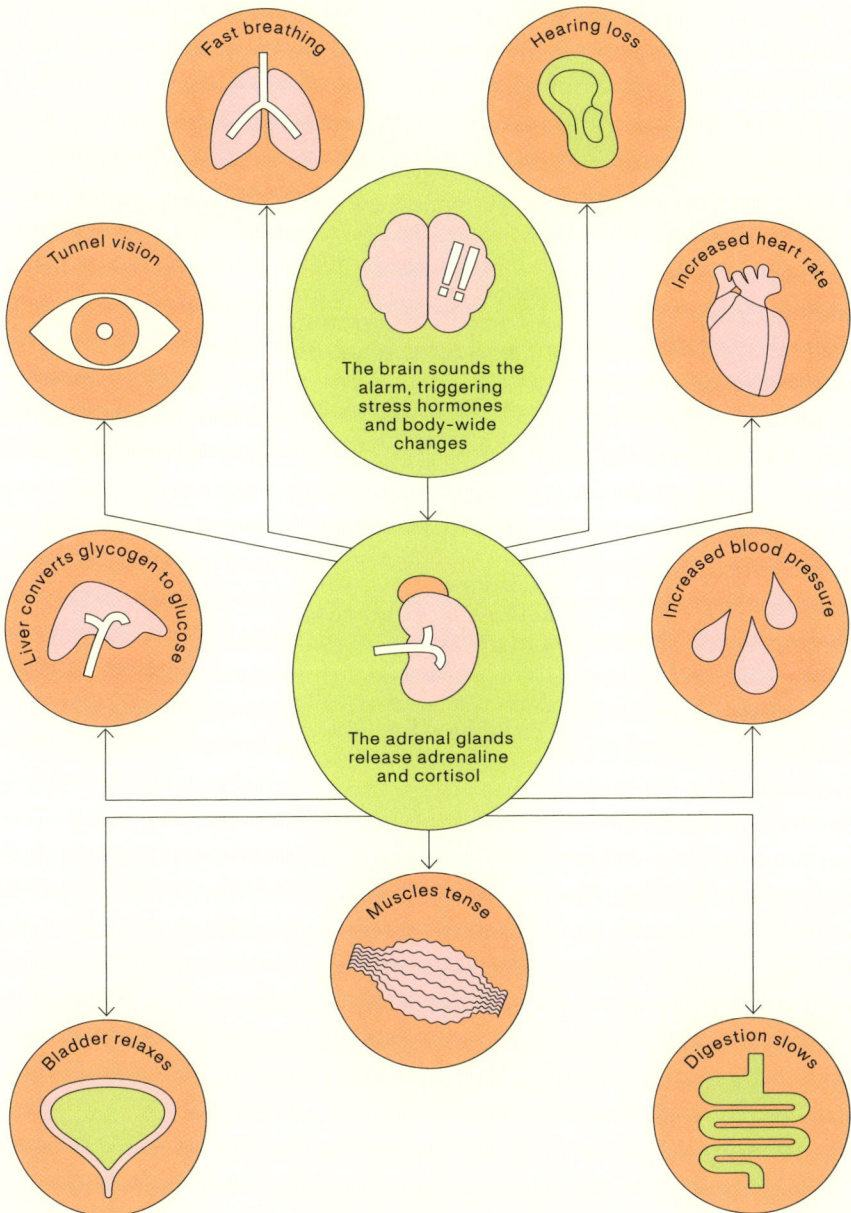

THE STRESS-RESPONSE SYSTEM
When we feel stress or alarm, the brain responds by triggering the "fight or flight" response by releasing adrenaline and cortisol. These hormones have a number of effects on different areas of the body.

Fast breathing

Hearing loss

Tunnel vision

Increased heart rate

The brain sounds the alarm, triggering stress hormones and body-wide changes

Liver converts glycogen to glucose

Increased blood pressure

The adrenal glands release adrenaline and cortisol

Muscles tense

Bladder relaxes

Digestion slows

with significantly steady or blunted levels of cortisol throughout the day are more likely to experience depression than those with diurnal cortisol curve patterns. A "flatlined" daily cortisol pattern, on the other hand, can indicate a dysfunctional stress response or even be linked to childhood trauma, and is as much of an issue as one that is off the charts.

The evidence drives home just how important it is to maintain a healthy diurnal rhythm for both physical and mental wellbeing, something we'll explore in more detail in Pillar Six (see p.195).

MEASURING CORTISOL: LOW OR HIGH?

When measuring your cortisol levels, a simple blood test only shows your "free" cortisol; it's a time stamp of one point in your day, and won't provide the whole picture. By contrast, saliva tests taken throughout the day can reveal much more. You can even try to run a sense check with yourself, seeing how you feel at different points throughout the day.

Although numerous issues arise from high cortisol – it's often what I see in clinic – many issues are also rooted in rhythm. What does low cortisol look like? The answer, quite often, is fatigue.

Research shows that low "free" cortisol may be linked to a suboptimal stress response due to poor brain signalling or gland dysfunction. This is a more likely theory than thinking that your adrenal glands have simply been overworked and given up (you may have heard of the expression "adrenal fatigue"). Adrenal fatigue is therefore less likely about tired adrenals and more related to suboptimal stress response.

GLUCOCORTICOIDS

Cortisol is a glucocorticoid, an anti-inflammatory steroid hormone that affects metabolism and the immune system. It can increase abdominal fat by storing it around the organs and also boost cravings for high-fat, sugary foods. This is a survival response, as the body historically stored fat to protect itself during threats like famine.

High cortisol can drive high androgens, which will have a knock-on effect on oestrogen and your ovulation – and therefore on your progesterone as well. High cortisol can also have a direct impact on your oestrogen levels, driving oestrogen deficiency in women of all ages.

HIGH CORTISOL AND LOW OESTROGEN

Alongside your HPA axis, there's also something called your HPO (hypothalamic-pituitary-ovarian) axis.

During highly stressful moments, we can end up entering into a state called functional hypothalamic amenorrhoea – when your HPO axis stops communicating. When this complex communication pathway comes to a halt and is suppressed, it's one of the leading issues for young premenopausal women suffering from low oestrogen.

Women in their prime reproductive years should have an abundance of oestrogen, but we are seeing increasingly inadequate levels that can compromise health. Given how important oestrogen is for overall wellbeing (see p.32), prolonged low levels can increase the risk of metabolic syndrome, which can lead to obesity, type 2 diabetes, and certain cancers such as colon cancer.

The drop in oestrogen levels during menopause brings risks related to your cardiovascular system, bone health, and psychological health. So, do these same risks apply to premenopausal women with low oestrogen? The answer is a resounding yes. And on top of this, low oestrogen during your most fertile years can compromise your reproductive system. Research shows that young premenopausal women experiencing low oestrogen due to functional hypothalamic amenorrhea – estimated to affect about 1.62 million women between the ages of 18 and 44 years in the US and 17.4 million women worldwide – experience issues that include missed periods, abnormal vascular function, premature cardiovascular disease, bone loss, and increased anxiety and depression.

These are symptoms and health risks typically seen in perimenopause and menopause, now appearing in young women as a result of elevated cortisol.

This review made another very important point: many women are not aware of the link between high stress and their health. Often, young women do not seek help when they experience menstrual irregularities, and when they do, they're frequently dismissed.

This science now links high stress to lower progesterone levels, which questions the "cortisol steal" theory which posits that, when the body is under stress, it prioritizes cortisol production over progesterone.

CORTISOL AND INSULIN RESISTANCE

There is a strong link between elevated cortisol levels and the risk of insulin resistance. Where an individual faces high levels of stress, symptoms of insulin resistance are often apparent, such as excess fat storage around the midsection. This abdominal weight gain includes subcutaneous fat (just below your skin) and visceral fat (deeper within the abdominal cavity, surrounding your organs).

Cortisol is also linked to your blood sugar. In the liver, high cortisol levels increase gluconeogenesis (when the body creates glucose – "neo" meaning new, "genesis" meaning creation). This metabolizes your glucose reserves for energy, and plonks it into your bloodstream. This means that stress can drive a glucose spike to supply energy for whatever danger you are facing. If you need to run for your life, your body will ensure that you can.

If your sources of stress are more psychological – perhaps you're about to deliver a big presentation, or an unpleasant email has just landed in your inbox – and less about fighting off wild animals, where does that excess energy go? It is stored as fat, particularly around your waist. Restricting food and over-exercising to counteract this can backfire, raising cortisol levels. This stress makes your body hold onto fat, outsmarting your efforts. Without calming your nervous system, long-term results are unlikely.

Women have been shown to experience a cycle where stress can lead to increased belly fat. Where there is more stress, there can be more abdominal fat, and where there is more abdominal fat, there may be higher cortisol production. One study investigating whether women with central fat distribution (as indicated by a high waist-to-hip ratio across a range of body mass indexes) display consistently

CHRONIC STRESS RESPONSE

Chronic stress progresses from a normal response (heightened alertness) to resistance (adaptation to ongoing pressure), and finally to exhaustion (burnout and fatigue).

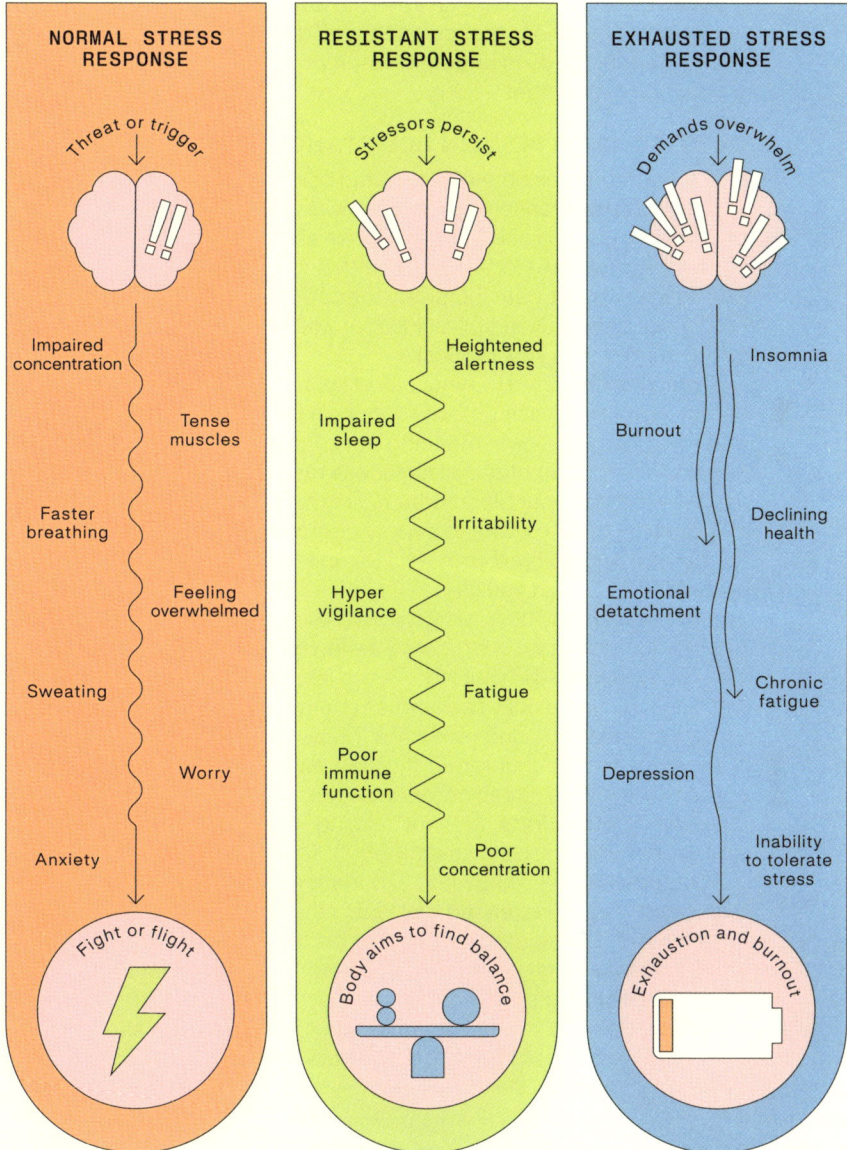

NORMAL STRESS RESPONSE

Threat or trigger

Impaired concentration

Tense muscles

Faster breathing

Feeling overwhelmed

Sweating

Worry

Anxiety

Fight or flight

RESISTANT STRESS RESPONSE

Stressors persist

Heightened alertness

Impaired sleep

Irritability

Hyper vigilance

Fatigue

Poor immune function

Poor concentration

Body aims to find balance

EXHAUSTED STRESS RESPONSE

Demands overwhelm

Insomnia

Burnout

Declining health

Emotional detatchment

Chronic fatigue

Depression

Inability to tolerate stress

Exhaustion and burnout

DAILY FREE CORTISOL
When operating as they should, cortisol levels peak in the morning, decline throughout the day, and reach their lowest point at night.

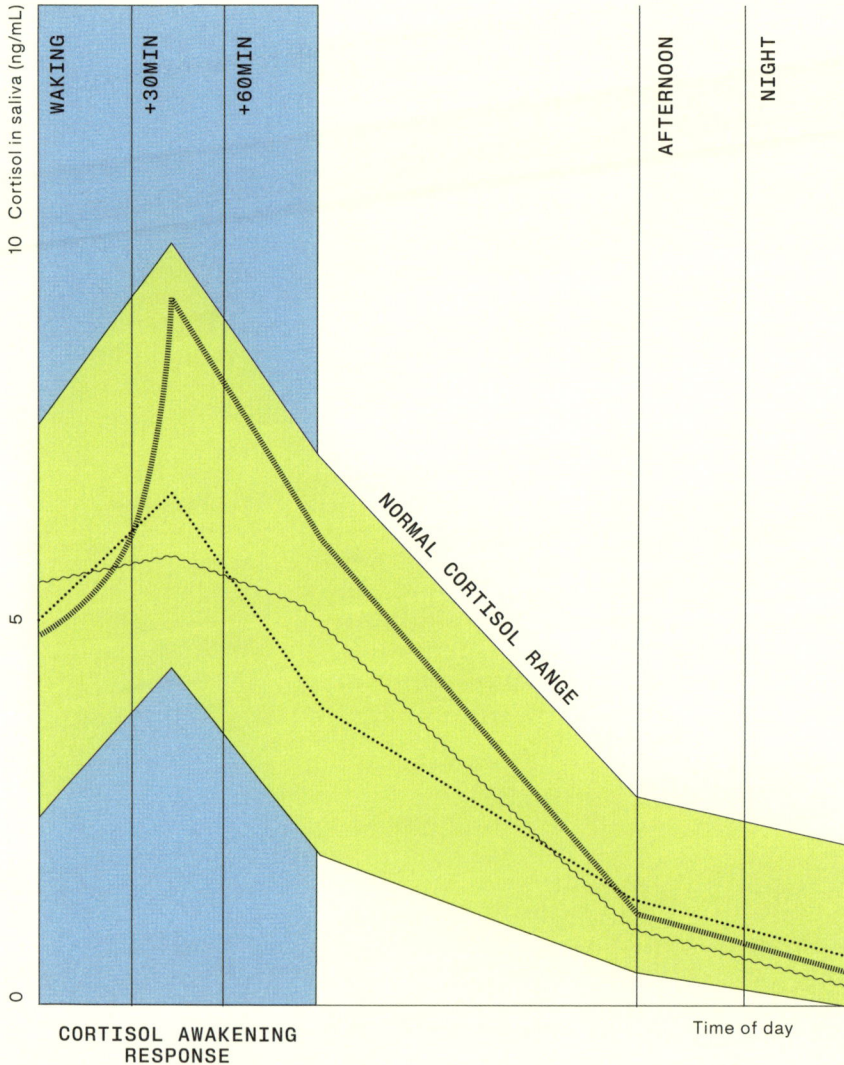

Cortisol in saliva (ng/mL)

10

5

0

WAKING

+30MIN

+60MIN

AFTERNOON

NIGHT

NORMAL CORTISOL RANGE

CORTISOL AWAKENING RESPONSE

Time of day

.... Ideal cortisol awakening response

～～～～～～ Low cortisol awakening response

|||||||||||||||||||||||||| Elevated cortisol awakening response

heightened cortisol reactivity to repeated laboratory stressors. It concluded that central fat distribution is related to greater psychological vulnerability to stress and cortisol reactivity. The current cross-sectional findings support the hypothesis that stress-induced cortisol secretion may contribute to central fat, and demonstrates a link between psychological stress and risk for disease.

WHAT DOES ELEVATED CORTISOL LOOK LIKE?*

Weight gain in face or waistline	Acne
Low appetite in the morning	Back fat deposit
Thinning hair	

CORTISOL: THE BIG PICTURE

What are the most common drivers and mediators of high cortisol? These issues are deep-rooted and systemic for women today, on a global scale. While unique to the individual, many aspects of being a women, at any age, come with pressures and pitfalls that can leave us feeling overwhelmed. Whether it's struggling with a lack of sleep, trying to balance work with life or being a mother, providing care, meeting deadlines, preparing for exams, navigating social media, being gaslit by doctors, or navigating toxic relationships – stressors are constant.

Cortisol, while essential for short-term stress, can become permanently elevated when dealing with ongoing pressures like these, leading to anxiety and burnout. While we cannot change the wild nature of life, we can support the nervous system and bring down elevated cortisol, lightening some of life's burdens. In chapter 3, you will experience something truly transformative as you learn to nurture and nourish your nervous system and rewrite your personal narrative.

*symptoms include, but are not limited to, this list

Insulin

Insulin is the gatekeeper, energy storage manager, and the lock and key to glucose regulation. When things are going well, insulin moves and stores energy-rich substrates like glucose into your liver, your muscles, and fat tissue.It's produced by your pancreas in response to glucose entering your bloodstream from either high-glucose foods or a stress-induced glucose release from your liver, helping to restore a steady amount of glucose in your bloodstream by removing any excess.

INSULIN'S JOURNEY

Glucose usually enters the bloodstream after you have eaten simple sugars or starchy carbohydrates, once they are broken down into glucose molecules. These molecules go on to be converted into adenosine triphosphate (ATP), the energy source of our cells. Insulin's crucial role is not only helping to store energy, but also preventing excessive levels of glucose in your blood. When you eat food, your body breaks it down into a currency that can be spent within the body. When you consume carbohydrates, for instance, they are broken down into starch, then into glucose which is used to produce ATP. This will be covered in more detail in Pillar One (see p.125).

Too much glucose in your bloodstream is dangerous. Just like the brakes in your car, insulin is there for a reason, stepping in to quickly bring glucose spikes under control when needed.

When you experience a glucose spike, it means that too much glucose has entered your bloodstream at any one time. This might be because of something you have eaten, or moments of stress.

MONITORING INSULIN

Glucose regulation – like cortisol – is a hot topic. This regulation works through a negative feedback loop, where rising glucose levels trigger insulin release, and once glucose is lowered, insulin secretion decreases to maintain balance.

It's important to remember, though, that glucose spikes are a normal part of your body's daily biological processes.

NEGATIVE FEEDBACK SYSTEM
A negative feedback loop is a self-regulating
biological system. It is a mechanism that uses
a system's output to regulate or reduce its own
activity to maintain homeostasis, which is the
optimal internal state of the body. The body uses
negative feedback loops to regulate blood sugar,
temperature, pH, and hormone levels.

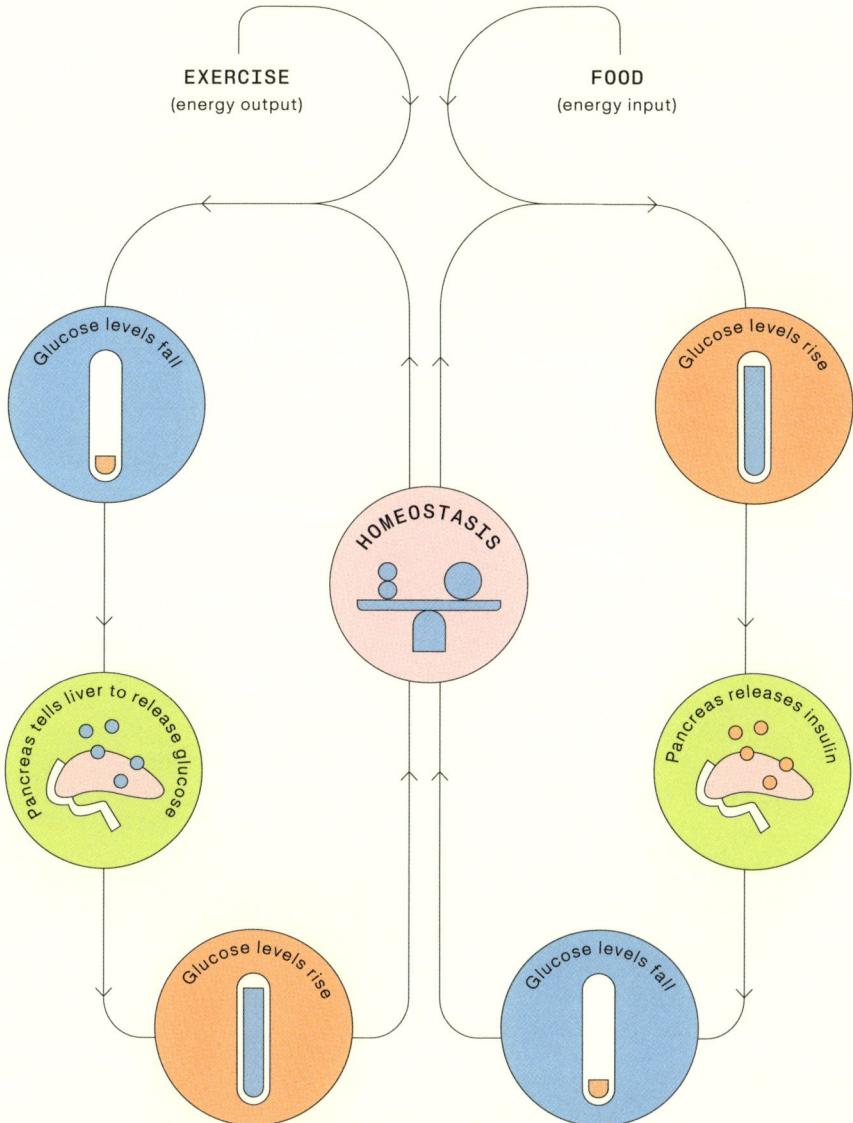

EXERCISE
(energy output)

FOOD
(energy input)

Glucose levels fall

Glucose levels rise

HOMEOSTASIS

Pancreas tells liver to release glucose

Pancreas releases insulin

Glucose levels rise

Glucose levels fall

It's why we have insulin in our bodies in the first place: to manage and regulate glucose spikes.

Glucose monitors may be the wellness accessory of the moment, but I'm uncertain about their benefits for non-diabetic individuals. Without the guidance of a medical professional, they can open a Pandora's box of data that quickly becomes overwhelming.

WHERE'S THE DANGER?

There's no need to fear insulin or glucose themselves. What you *should* watch out for is excess – whether that's excess glucose, excess simple sugars, excess insulin, or excess cortisol. Excess insulin or glucose can create a disease-prone inflammatory environment for your body, directly impacting how your hormones work together.

Relying on insulin to mop up a sugary mess numerous times a day will put a lot of pressure on your system. If insulin is popping up in your bloodstream and lingering, it can cause high blood pressure and increase fat creation in your liver (lipogenesis), which could drive non-alcoholic fatty liver disease.

When your body becomes less efficient at responding to insulin, insulin resistance can hinder glucose by preventing the body's cells from taking in glucose effectively. This means that you cannot properly create energy from glucose, causing you to feel completely drained even though your body is loaded with potential energy from sugar.

When insulin is called upon too often, it's like when brake pads start to wear down, leaving you with a car that is unsafe to drive. If you push this mechanism to the limit, your hormone health – not to mention your overall health – will be compromised.

Insulin isn't just about blood sugar; it is the gatekeeper to your hormone and metabolic health. Insulin resistance plays a critical role in the development of endocrine disorders, in particular excess androgens (like your male sexual characteristic hormones, such as testosterone). When insulin resistance and high androgen levels create a vicious cycle, they can aggravate each other. Insulin resistance can trigger increased androgen production, with higher androgen levels creating a feedback loop (see p.67) that disrupts metabolic and hormonal balance.

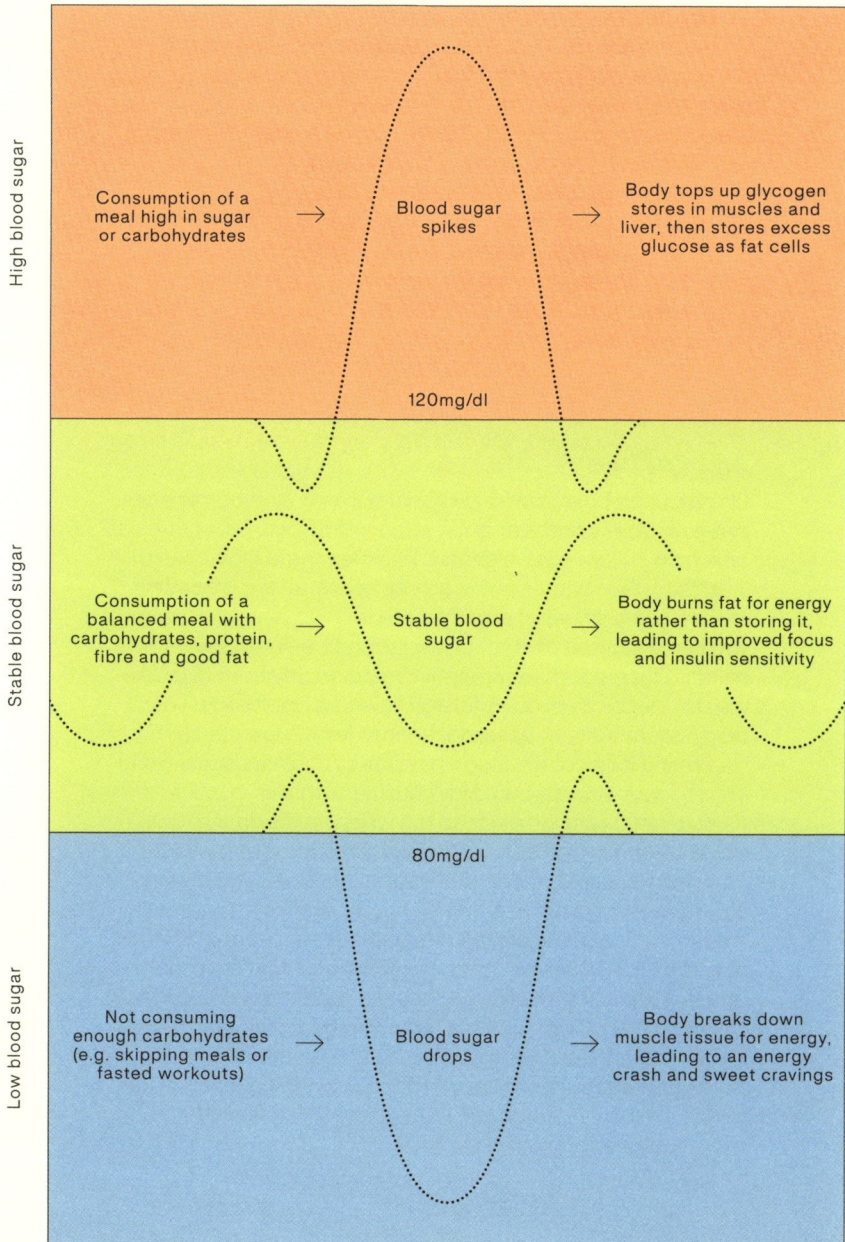

BLOOD SUGAR
Blood sugar can often spike after eating, stabilize with the help of insulin, and then drop during fasting or intense activity.

High blood sugar

Consumption of a meal high in sugar or carbohydrates → Blood sugar spikes → Body tops up glycogen stores in muscles and liver, then stores excess glucose as fat cells

120mg/dl

Stable blood sugar

Consumption of a balanced meal with carbohydrates, protein, fibre and good fat → Stable blood sugar → Body burns fat for energy rather than storing it, leading to improved focus and insulin sensitivity

80mg/dl

Low blood sugar

Not consuming enough carbohydrates (e.g. skipping meals or fasted workouts) → Blood sugar drops → Body breaks down muscle tissue for energy, leading to an energy crash and sweet cravings

HOW DOES INSULIN WORK?

When too much glucose enters into your bloodstream, the pancreas releases insulin, which acts like a key, unlocking cells to allow glucose to be stored. Hormones operate in a targeted way, and insulin has one goal: to keep your blood glucose levels in check.

The first stops are your muscles and liver. Insulin allows glucose to enter these cells, rapidly moving it out of your bloodstream and into your muscles to be stored as energy – until your muscles reach capacity, that is. Your muscles only have so much room to store glucose as energy, and it's highly dependent on your muscle mass. Insulin stores any leftover glucose as fat, often as visceral fat around your middle. Unfortunately, there's an infinite amount of storage space for glucose in the form of fat cells.

INSULIN IN OVERDRIVE

Once the glucose is well and truly out of your bloodstream, insulin's job is done – or is it?

Insulin can do such a great job of clearing out glucose that it ends up removing all of it, storing away all the glucose and leaving you drained of energy.

The spike then plummets, and you experience something called a low blood sugar dip – the crash after the high. As well as feeling zapped of energy, this can involve low mood, brain fog, fatigue, and feeling 'hangry', which is just your body screaming for more glucose to extend the high. During a blood sugar dip, you'll also burn lean muscle – not fat.

Your brain runs on glucose, so when levels drop, it signals you to seek out more. This explains why sweet cravings tend to kick in around 11 am and 3 pm, and during those post-dinner hours.

If we continue on this roller coaster, our cells are eventually unable to communicate with one another. They begin resisting the insulin that's meant to be managing the glucose spikes, so that more insulin is needed to manage blood sugar levels. The end result is that your body becomes less sensitive to insulin, which we call insulin resistance (see p.99).

Your Thyroid

The thyroid gland plays a pivotal role in the regulation of your metabolism. It monitors the body's energy needs and releases hormones accordingly, ensuring that every cell receives the necessary signals to function efficiently. The hormones produced from this gland are essential for mitochondrial metabolism, often referred to as your body's energy factories.

The butterfly-shaped thyroid gland produces the hormones T3 (triiodothyronine – the active thyroid hormone) and T4 (thyroxine – the non-active thyroid hormone). Your pituitary gland then produces thyroid-stimulating hormone (TSH), which regulates T4 and T3. These two hormones control everything from your heartbeat and appetite to your temperature.

THYROID DYSFUNCTION

As we age, the risk of thyroid dysfunction increases. The diagnosis for hypothyroidism, which is when your pituitary gland produces too much thyroid-stimulating hormone, is solely based on blood reference ranges. This can overlook subclinical states where thyroid function is still impaired. For example, if your T4 is normal but your TSH is slightly elevated, current guidelines may label your results as "normal", and no action will be taken. You may have early signs of an underactive thyroid, but your results don't meet the diagnostic criteria. Thyroid issues can therefore go undetected. If there is an issue, it will fall into one of two camps: underactive or overactive.

UNDERACTIVE THYROID

Thyroid hormone deficiency can be described as hypothyroidism, indicated by high levels of TSH and low levels of T4 and T3. The absence of adequate thyroid hormones can lead to a sluggish metabolism, and can present as weight gain, fertility issues, hair loss, feeling cold, poor hearing, slow heart rate, poor memory, fatigue, and low mood.

A lack of thyroid hormones can lead to overt hypothyroidism, which is commonly driven by iodine deficiency, or could indicate an autoimmune condition, such as Hashimoto's thyroiditis. This disorder causes the immune system to attack the thyroid gland, reducing hormone production and leading to hypothyroidism. It triggers a chronic reaction by attacking thyroid antigens.

OVERACTIVE THYROID

Hyperthyroidism sits at the other end of the spectrum. It is relatively rare and often linked to an autoimmune condition such as Graves' disease or benign thyroid nodules that overproduce thyroid hormone.

The excess thyroid hormones then overstimulate the metabolism, typically presenting as rapid heart rate, anxiety, tremors, irregular menstrual bleeding, and weight loss.

HYPOTHYROIDISM

Hypothyroidism will present with high TSH secretion, and can be driven by low thyrotropin-releasing hormone (TRH) from the hypothalamus, poor conversion of T4 to T3, or inefficient thyroid hormone utilisation. Iodine deficiency is also a major cause – certain foods can actually interfere with iodine absorption.

Diagnosis should be confirmed by a doctor, but your basal body temperature can offer clues. To support your thyroid health, increase your intake of iodine, iron, selenium, tyrosine, and copper.

Hypothyroidism plays out on a spectrum. Many women would be considered to have subclinical hypothyroidism, but their blood results are not in the precise reference range. That's not to say these women are not experiencing the symptoms, though!

Serotonin

Time to smile, as we come to your happy neurotransmitter. Serotonin begins life with the essential amino acid tryptophan, made predominantly in your gut, specifically in your enterochromaffin cells found in the gut lining. These cells release serotonin to help regulate digestion and communicate with the brain. Some serotonin is also created in the raphe nuclei, a cluster of nuclei found in the brain stem.

You may have heard serotonin referred to as your "happy hormone", and this is because the biggest role it plays is in your central nervous system. It can affect and stabilize your mood, and also plays a role in memory, sleep, motor skills, wound healing, anger, fear, appetite, stress, addiction, sexual function, pleasure and pain perception, cerebral vascular tone, and your central respiratory system.

SEROTONIN, DOPAMINE, AND MOOD DISORDERS

What differentiates dopamine from serotonin? Dopamine is a neurotransmitter produced in the brain that regulates mood, motivation, pleasure, and reward, and controls movement, learning, and attention. Serotonin, meanwhile, is synthesized from the amino acid tryptophan, highlighting its distinct role in mood and wellbeing.

NEUROTRANSMITTERS

A neurotransmitter is a chemical messenger that carries information between nerve cells, muscles, and glands in the body. Serotonin acts as both a neurotransmitter and a hormone, affecting mood and cognition in the brain and regulating digestion and other processes in the body. Hormones can wear several hats and serve multiple additional functions, as antioxidants, neurotransmitters, and more.

DOPAMINE	SEROTONIN
produced mainly in your brain	produced mainly in your gut
makes you feel more alert	encourages better sleep
drives your motivation and reward response	stabilizes your mood and happiness

Recent research has shown that serotonin also plays a role in your metabolism, enhancing nutrient absorption and storage, and even prompting movement in the gut through a series of wave-like muscle contractions. This process is triggered when glucose and fatty acids are present, signalling serotonin to get your digestion moving.

Serotonin is another neurotransmitter that drops during the perimenopause. Oestrogen and progesterone both have an effect on serotonin, and the tailspin of declining hormonal fluctuations during the perimenopause can also drive a drop in serotonin. This can trigger mood disorders during the perimenopause, menopause, and postmenopause. The SWAN study looking into national data across the US over 10 years found that the risk for high depressive symptoms and disorder is greater during and possibly after menopause.

Serotonin's finely tuned responses serve as a reminder to never take hormones at face value; they usually have a number of other functions up their sleeve.

Melatonin

Melatonin is the hormone in charge of your bedtime. More than just a sleepy hormone, melatonin is created in the pineal gland, and its secretion occurs in response to darkness in the evening. I call it your vampire hormone – it loves the dark. As well as playing a critical role in your sleep cycle, it protects and supports your ovarian functions including ovulation, follicular development, luteal function, and egg maturation. Insufficient levels of melatonin can be linked to the underlying causes of many endocrine disorders.

If your sleep at night or alertness during the day feels off, or if fertility is important for you, it's vital that you harness the positive power of this hormone, which has strong antioxidant properties.

MELATONIN'S JOURNEY

There are four steps involved in melatonin's creation. Tryptophan is first converted into 5-hydroxytryptophan, which then becomes serotonin. Serotonin is then converted into N-acetylserotonin, which is converted into melatonin. The whole process happens in your gut, all thanks to a protein called tryptophan and the cells in your gut.

MITOCHONDRIA

Your mitochondria are small, membrane-bound structures within cells that perform a specific function – they are your energy powerhouses. They create energy via a series of chemical reactions required for the cell's survival and functioning. Your mitochondria break down glucose into an energy molecule known as adenosine triphosphate (ATP). They are the factories behind your energy – and melatonin is out to protect them at all costs.

We call these your enterochromaffin cells. They are a type of endocrine cell in the gut lining that produce serotonin and melatonin. They release both of these hormones onto nearby sensory nerve endings. These cells also modulate intestinal function and movement, and they can also detect environmental and internal stimuli that may enter the gut such as dietary irritants, inflammatory agents, and stress hormones.

The denser your enterochromaffin cells in your gut, the better your distribution of melatonin!

MELATONIN AND CIRCADIAN RHYTHM

While melatonin triggers sleepiness in a dark environment, cortisol triggers your get-up-and-go in the morning, waking you up. These two hormones are the key ingredients to a healthy circadian rhythm. Disturbances in your circadian rhythm can be associated with other hormonal imbalances and chronic diseases such as insomnia, high blood pressure, diabetes, and depression.

Melatonin can impact your hormonal balance because it regulates many biological functions, including circadian rhythm, immunity, reproduction and, of course, sleep. All of these factors impact the environment for your hormones. Bad sleep equals bad hormone function, which we will discuss in Pillar Five (see p.184) when we learn how to improve the quality of your sleep.

MELATONIN AND MITOCHONDRIA

Melatonin is also an incredible antioxidant. An antioxidant works by mopping up damage from free radicals in the body. Antioxidants protect the body by neutralizing free radicals, unstable molecules formed during normal processes such as metabolism, as well as from environmental toxins (like pollution, UV rays, cigarette smoke) and unhealthy diets.

Melatonin is a free radical scavenger, which means that it has the power to neutralize harmful free radicals in the body. This comes with bonus anti-inflammatory effects. Melatonin has an antioxidant effect on your reproductive system, as well as for your mitochondria (the factories for your energy production).

FREE RADICALS

A free radical is a molecule created in the body by certain foods, types of exercise, or exposure to toxins. They contain one or more unpaired electrons. This odd number makes it unstable and highly reactive. When free radicals outnumber your antioxidants, it can lead to oxidative stress.

Numerous studies have confirmed that melatonin can protect key mitochondrial components, such as proteins in the electron transport chain and the mitochondrial genome. Melatonin specifically targets the mitochondria, and seems to function as their protector, shielding them from free radicals.

Oxytocin

Oxytocin, fondly known as the love hormone, is a peptide hormone and neuropeptide normally produced in the hypothalamus, where it is released by the pituitary gland. A peptide hormone is a small chain of amino acids that helps regulate various bodily functions, while a neuropeptide is a signalling molecule in the nervous system that influences communication between nerve cells and affects processes like mood and pain perception. Oxytocin is also called the bonding or kindness hormone. When your brain releases dopamine, your serotonin levels go up and oxytocin is produced. Alongside these neurotransmitters, it's part of the feel-good family.

Oxytocin triggers labour and breastmilk production, as well as strengthening the parental bond. It also enhances positive memories, feelings of safety, decision-making, empathy, trust, fidelity, and communication. Oxytocin supports your immune system, enhancing the production of immunoglobulin – vital for your immune function. It's even associated with the big O, increasing and enhancing pleasure during the female orgasm.

I like to refer to oxytocin as cortisol's kryptonite; oxytocin can inhibit the stress-induced activity of your HPA axis and promote the return of normal cortisol levels. Therefore, the more oxytocin you make, the more efficiently cortisol can be lowered after a stressful situation. Where there are low levels of oxytocin, research has shown an increase in stress, anxiety, and even hormonal disorders like PCOS.

OXYTOCIN AND MENOPAUSE

As perimenopause begins, oxytocin levels gradually decline. This decrease has been linked to menopause-related risks, including cardiovascular disease, osteoporosis, urinary incontinence, sexual dysfunction, obesity, and low metabolism.

Oxytocin is a tonic that women of all ages, but particularly those in later years, should be increasing as eventually its levels naturally begin to decline. Oxytocin has the power to reduce cortisol, and boost happiness and health. How can we increase oxytocin? We'll get to that in Pillar Six (see p.195).

FSH and LH

Before we get into the mechanics of hormones in action, let's meet FSH and LH. Made from comparable genes, FSH and LH have similar properties but are in charge of different mechanisms.

Follicle-stimulating hormone (FSH) is a hormone produced by your pituitary gland in response to gonadotropin-releasing hormone (GnRH) from the hypothalamus. It regulates the function of your ovaries, peaking midway through your cycle to stimulate the maturation of eggs during the follicular phase. It also promotes the enzyme called aromatase, which is in charge of converting testosterone to oestradiol.

Luteinizing hormone (LH) is a glycoprotein hormone that is co-secreted along with follicle-stimulating hormone by your pituitary gland. This hormone prompts the ovulation and release of an egg, as well as the secretion of progesterone.

As you enter into the perimenopause, FSH starts to elevate in response to the drop in oestrogen. As FSH peaks, so too does LH. These hormones work with oestrogen and progesterone through a negative feedback system.

Your Endocrine System

Now that we've met the main hormones we'll be dealing with, let's pause for a quick recap. Hormones are the chemical messengers that create a cascade of effects impacting nearly every aspect of your body and your behaviour. From metabolism, energy, growth, and development to reproduction, sexual function, mood, blood sugar levels, and stress – name the bodily function, and you can make a safe bet that hormones are involved. That explains why they are linked to such a wide range of symptoms.

So, how do these hormones go about their business? The simple answer is, via your endocrine system. This is a network of glands that produce and release hormones into your bloodstream and tissues. These glands include your hypothalamus, pituitary, pineal, thyroid, and thymus, as well as the endocrine portion of the pancreas, four parathyroid glands, two adrenal glands, and your ovaries. None of these glands are physically connected, but they are all able to communicate with one another through a negative feedback system, ensuring your body stays within a normal range when everything is balanced. However, when this balance is disrupted – whether by illness, lifestyle factors, or other issues – it can lead to dysfunction.

WHY HORMONE BALANCE MATTERS
Think of your hormones like salt granules dissolved in water: they're present, but invisible. Once secreted, they travel through the body, delivering specific chemical messages. This process can be broken down into four phases. Each of these phases can be negatively or positively influenced by diet, lifestyle, and environmental factors. A problem in just one of these phases can have powerful consequences.

THE FOUR STEPS OF HORMONE FUNCTION (AND DYSFUNCTION)

STEP ONE: PRODUCTION OF YOUR HORMONES

Hormones must be successfully secreted by a gland. Are you making too much or too little of a hormone, and is it happening at the right time? Do you have the nutrients and building blocks to create your hormones? Is the negative feedback system working?

STEP TWO: TRANSPORTATION OF YOUR HORMONES

Hormones must travel through your bloodstream to reach their target cell. Is the transport system working? Do you have poor circulation? Are your hormones able to get to their destination, or are they turning up somewhere else and causing mischief?

STEP THREE: RECEPTION OF YOUR HORMONES

When hormones deliver their messages they set off a cascade of change. Is the message getting through? Is there another, more potent hormone blocking the way? Have the receptors been damaged? Are your target receptors able to pick up the messages sent by your hormones? This is what we call functional hormone resistance, which is like your receptors becoming less responsive.

STEP FOUR: DETOXIFICATION

This is how your hormones are metabolized and cleared out of your body. Are your hormones being broken down and optimally disposed of, or is there a build-up of hormones that should have left your system?

THE JOURNEY HORMONES TAKE AROUND THE BODY

A hormone's journey, from secretion to detoxification, is a quest of epic proportions. Much of its time is spent cruising the highways of your bloodstream on a mission to find its target cell.

As blood is water-based, any fat-based hormones (such as oestrogen, testosterone, and cortisol) must bind onto a transportation protein synthesized by the liver. If there is no such transportation protein available, these hormones are considered "free". Oestrogen and testosterone bind to sex hormone-binding globulins (SHBG for short) and cortisol binds to cortisol-binding globulin (CBG), also known as transcortin and albumin.

Once secreted, these hormones hop onto their SHBG or CBG (just like you might get onto a bus) and head off on their journey with one goal in mind: to reach their target cell and deliver their message.

WHEN THE JOURNEY IS DISRUPTED

What happens if there's a disruption to the hormone's journey through the body? Imagine rush hour in a big city. Buses and cars head in every direction every minute. All of a sudden, all transportation is reduced to running every hour. What would happen? A backlog would form pretty rapidly.

In the body, this backlog represents an accumulation of "free" testosterone – testosterone that is not bound to sex hormone -binding globulins (SHBG). If there's no way out, this means that testosterone cannot bind to SHBG, which not only transports it from A to B, but also controls how much "active" testosterone is available by preventing tissues from using it immediately. We then see testosterone levels increasing, just as we might see a crowd growing as it waits for a reduced bus service.

What reduces the transportation system around your body? The answer is insulin resistance.

HOW DO HORMONES COMMUNICATE?

Each hormone interacts and binds with its own target cell through receptors uniquely recognized by that hormone. Only cells with the appropriate receptors can receive and respond to the hormone's signal, ensuring precise communication and biological regulation. Only certain keys will fit certain locks, as it were! This moment of "docking" is called "the reception". Visualize a square hormone only being able to deliver a message into a square receptor, and a star-shaped hormone travelling past any square-shaped receptors until it finds its target cell with a star-shaped receptor. Once found, they fit like a glove. If it's not the right fit, that hormone won't be able to mediate that cell and the cascade will not be initiated. If it's the correct target, a hormone will then mediate changes in the target cell. This sets off a pathway, initiating a modification to that cell.

This interaction is called a "receptor complex". It presents itself as a behaviour or a physiological change in your body. Once the cascade has finished, the function of that cell has finished. You then bid goodbye to that hormone, which is destroyed or detoxified via the liver.

HOW DYSFUNCTION OCCURS

Dysfunction can occur at each step. Another, more potent hormone, like cortisol, could be blocking the receptors. Big, powerful cortisol can dock in and block other hormones from delivering a message. While cortisol is vital, too much of it can create a metabolic disaster.

There is a root cause driving each of your symptoms, which we will identify and address to change the narrative, creating a more favourable environment for your hormones. Once we pinpoint what is driving your symptoms, we can set the cogs in motion for true, sustainable change.

PCOS Typically high androgens, insulin, cortisol, low oestrogen, serotonin, and melatonin

Endometriosis Typically high oestrogen, progesterone, resistance

Hypothyroidism Typically high TSH, low free thyroxine

Perimenopause/Menopause Declining oestrogen, progesterone, testosterone, serotonin, and higher risk of insulin resistance

HOW DO HORMONES COMMUNICATE?

Hormones communicate by docking onto specific receptors on target cells, triggering a response that regualtes bodily functions and behaviour.

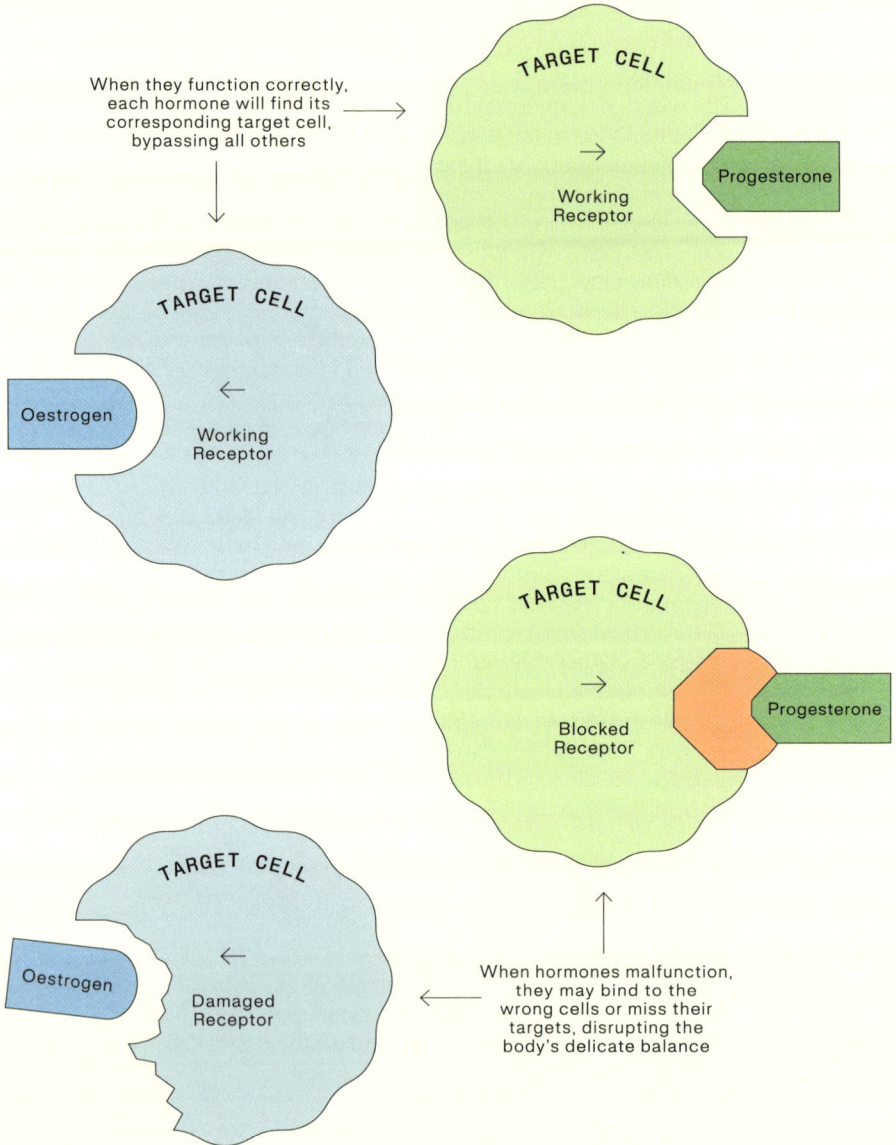

When they function correctly, each hormone will find its corresponding target cell, bypassing all others

TARGET CELL

→

Working Receptor

Progesterone

TARGET CELL

←

Oestrogen

Working Receptor

TARGET CELL

→

Blocked Receptor

Progesterone

TARGET CELL

←

Oestrogen

Damaged Receptor

When hormones malfunction, they may bind to the wrong cells or miss their targets, disrupting the body's delicate balance

The Intricate Dance of Hormones

The world of hormones is a bit incestuous. Testosterone, as we learned earlier, is a precursor hormone to oestrogen. Another important hormone duo is serotonin and melatonin. Serotonin (your happy neurotransmitter) is the precursor to your sleep hormone melatonin. If this has you feeling a little confused, don't worry, it certainly can be. Our bodies are incredibly resourceful in their processes – and hormone synthesis is no different.

As you can see in the hormone creation pathway on p.30, progesterone and cortisol both come from pregnenolone. One theory, often called the "cortisol or pregnenolone steal", links high stress to low progesterone because, in stressful situations, your body will prioritize cortisol production – our survival hormone – over progesterone and other sex hormones. However, this doesn't account for the dizzying array of glands, enzymes, and pathways involved in sex hormone creation – there is no one pool of adrenal pregnenolone that cortisol can come and "steal" from.

As a circulating pro-hormone, testosterone can morph into oestrogen when needed. It can also convert into a levelled-up version of itself, becoming a potent androgen called DHT (5α-dihydrotesterone). This conversion is prompted by the enzyme 5α-reductase, whose activity can be increased by sleep deprivation and insulin resistance. Studies have shown 5α-reductase activity is enhanced in women with PCOS, highlighting the links to insulin resistance.

Thankfully, certain behaviours can also reduce this enzyme's activity, such as drinking green tea. We'll look at some others in Pillar Two (see p.137).

Hormones have intricate patterns of interaction, transforming into one another and ultimately impacting on another within a sophisticated set of pathways. That is why hormone health must be approached holistically.

TO RECAP

A gland secretes a hormone that travels to its specific target cell, where it delivers a message through receptors. After the message is received and a change occurs, the hormone is broken down by the target tissue or your liver, and then detoxified.

However, it's not always that simple. If you find yourself facing a hormonal shift, a life event, or an endocrine disorder, consider how you can honour your needs by creating an environment in which your hormones can thrive.

With the right diet and lifestyle, you can create an environment that allows your body to optimally play out all four phases of hormone function to the best of its ability.

Your Gut and Hormones

Your gastrointestinal tract accommodates your very own community of bacteria and fungi living within your gut – and we're talking trillions of them. Within this colony (known as the microbiata) lives a gene set estimated to total about 3 million genes – a whopping 150 times larger than that of the human genome. That's roughly 100 trillion microbes, representing as many as 5,000 different species and weighing approximately 2 kg (4.4 lb), which is heavier than your brain. It is the largest ecosystem in the human body.

THE GUT MICROBIOME

The microbes associated with your digestive tract are known as the gut microbiome. The gut microbiome is a vast subject, and one that has captured the attention of medical pioneers and researchers for decades. Over the last few years alone some seriously exciting discoveries have been made. What we know today still barely scratches the surface of this topic, and, with ongoing research, there's even more fascinating knowledge to be discovered on the horizon.

Your microbiome supports digestion, helps maintain mucosal integrity, and influences your psychological health via the gut-brain axis. Research highlights significant associations between gut health and cognitive function, suggesting that the gut microbiome composition can influence cognitive performance, too. It also impacts inflammation and your metabolism. Your gut is your immune system's first line of defence, and has a majority stake in your hormone health. A good gut will equal great hormones.

Like your thumbprint, your gut bacteria is completely unique to you. The bacteria and fungi residing there are living organisms influenced by almost everything – your diet, medication, and stress levels, the products and chemicals you're exposed to, and even where you live and who you live with – not to mention your hormonal environment. This means that you have the power to positively influence your gut microbiome.

DIGESTION: FROM THE MOUTH TO THE GUT

Digestion is a complex process involving the mouth, oesophagus, stomach, liver, pancreas, gallbladder, and intestines – all working together to break down food, absorb nutrients, and eliminate waste.

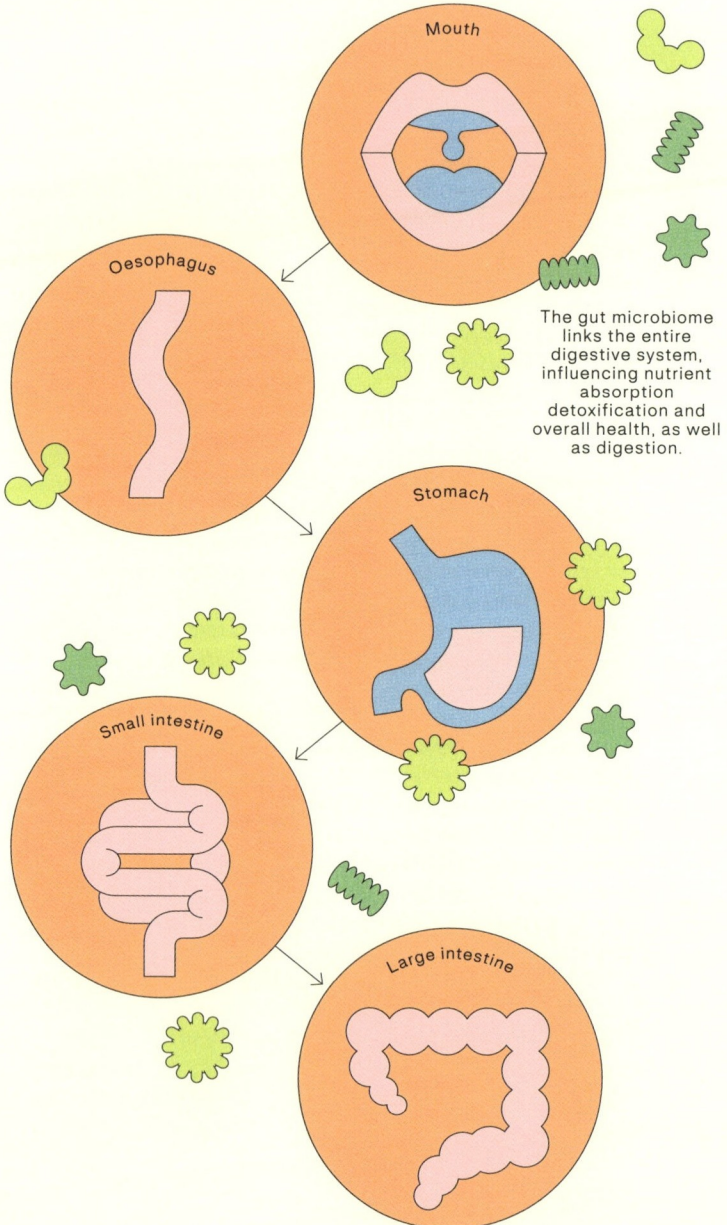

Mouth

Oesophagus

The gut microbiome links the entire digestive system, influencing nutrient absorption detoxification and overall health, as well as digestion.

Stomach

Small intestine

Large intestine

WHY IS YOUR GUT HEALTH SO IMPORTANT?

The gut microbiome is a community that can either thrive or become problematic. You can positively influence this community by maintaining gut diversity and healthy interactions. If neglected, an unhealthy hormonal balance could emerge – or even harmful microbes. In Pillar Three (see p.159), we'll learn how to populate, nourish, and feed a fabulous gut microbiome while boosting your nutrition.

If your community of bacteria and fungi is on the turn, it can look like an overgrowth of bad bacteria or fungi with limited and homogenous flora. The function of your endocrine system (see pp.80–83) can also be greatly compromised, particularly Step One (the secretion of hormones) and Step Four (the detoxification of hormones).

HORMONES AND YOUR GUT

The strongest connection between your gut and your hormones is with oestrogen, your life hormone. Specifically, it lies in oestrogen metabolism and the production of other important hormones such as serotonin and melatonin. While our understanding of the precise mechanisms between hormones and gut is still developing, we already know that the gut plays a central role in regulating circulating oestrogen levels. This balance is influenced by a collection of bacteria called the estrobolome.

While more research is needed to understand the complex relationship between hormones and the gut, what *is* clear is that your sex hormones – oestrogen, testosterone, progesterone, and cortisol– and your gut microbiome influence each other.

Recent studies have shown that individuals with PCOS tend to have a significantly lower diversity in their gut microbiome than that of individuals without the disorder. Another study identified six intestinal species which were present and characteristic markers for individuals with PCOS, highlighting a strong link between your hormones and your gut.

THE GUT AND YOUR OVERALL HEALTH

Supporting a diverse gut microbiome is a core part of maintaining your overall health. Where there are imbalances in the gut microbiome, there can be direct links to metabolic

ESTROBOLOME
Your estrobolome regulates oestrogen levels, influences
its circulation, and breaks it down for elimination or reactivation
in the body. It plays a key role in oestrogen clearance.

diseases, cancers, and autoimmune conditions. Add any
hormonal shifts or dysfunctions to the mix, and this becomes
a burden on your body that requires a gut in tip-top condition.

During the natural transition of perimenopause, supporting
a healthy gut is especially crucial due to one of the most
well-documented links between gut health and hormones
– gut health and oestrogen.

Research suggests that the drop in sex hormones during
the perimenopause and menopause, in particular the
decrease in oestradiol, is associated with reduced gut
microbiome diversity and a less active estrobolome. The
theory is that less oestrogen equals both less gut diversity
and an idle estrobolome, which perpetuates poor oestrogen
metabolism.

Gut imbalances and estrobolome dysfunction have been
linked to certain oestrogen-dependent diseases, including
endometriosis. It has also been linked to the development
and progression of hormone-dependent cancers, including
breast cancer.

YOUR ESTROBOLOME

One specific colony of microorganisms within the
microbiome worth our attention is known as the
estrobolome. This is a constellation of bacteria and gene-
encoding enzymes that influence both the excretion and
circulation of oestrogens. Like the broader gut microbiome,
its composition and function are shaped by factors such as
your diet, medication, and lifestyle, and can influence
ovulation, weight, libido, and mood. Emerging research
suggests that a woman's estrobolome plays a key role in a

number of hormonal disorders, as well as breast, endometrial, and ovarian cancers.

OESTROGEN CLEARANCE

Your estrobolome, along with your microflora, can influence oestrogen levels, which may in turn impact your weight, libido, and mood. To address this, we'll be giving your gut and estrobolome a helping hand – which is also going to support your vaginal microbiome.

Your estrobolome is where oestrogen bids its final farewell, after it passes through the liver for detoxification (see pp.94–95) and enters back into the gut, ready for excretion. Your gut and liver work in tandem to ensure the optimal clearance of oestrogen. If either system is compromised, you may not be able to remove oestrogen from your system at an optimal rate.

During detoxification, the liver deactivates oestrogen and changes its structure so that it is more water-soluble and can be excreted from the body. This process is called conjugation, which is the transformation of oestrogen to a highly water-soluble structure that we will cover in more detail on pp.96–97.

Oestrogen detoxification is strongly influenced by nutrition (see p.164) as the gut and liver directly drive this process. It's critical that we support oestrogen clearance, as otherwise we run the risk of oestrogen dominance and even oestrogen-dominant cancers.

WHEN OESTROGEN IS REACTIVATED

Once oestrogen is ready to leave your system, your gut may have other ideas. When estrobolome activity is impaired, gut dysbiosis (imbalance) increases circulating oestrogen. Your estrobolome has the power to reactivate oestrogen through deconjugation (the process of breaking down conjugated compounds). It does this via certain bacteria, along with beta-glucosidase activity, allowing oestrogen to be reabsorbed into the body. This leaves your body at risk of oestrogen excess.

Your Vaginal Microbiome

While most of us are familiar with the gut microbiome, the presence of the vaginal tract's own microbiome was identified just under a decade ago, and it remains the subject of ongoing research. While we are still in the early stages of research and understanding it, how we can influence and improve the vaginal microbiome holds great potential for gynaecologic and reproductive health. Watch this space!

A HEALTHY VAGINAL MICROBIOME?

Most of us are aware that a diverse gut flora is desirable, but the opposite is true for the vagina. A healthy vaginal flora is characterized by low diversity, primarily dominated by a species of bacteria called *Lactobacilli* – the same bacteria found in kefir and live yoghurt. This bacteria can thrive thanks to oestrogen, as glycogen production is aided by oestrogen, which is the main food source of the *Lactobacillus* species. This lactic acid-producing bacteria prevents the growth and spread of harmful pathogens, serving as a protective barrier and maintaining a balanced ecosystem. Having a colony rich in *Lactobacilli* will promote a beneficial acidic environment. The ideal balance is somewhere between pH 3.6 and 4.5.

A pH imbalance will be characterized by a disruption in your *Lactobacilli* colony. One example of this is bacterial vaginosis, where the vaginal environment becomes more alkaline as *Lactobacilli* levels decline. Maintaining the vaginal pH between 3.5 and 4.5 is a key protective barrier against pathogenic microorganisms – steer clear of any intimate washes that could disrupt this balance.

IMBALANCES IN THE VAGINAL MICROBIOME

The composition of your vaginal flora plays a major role in vaginal, reproductive, and overall health. An imbalance can trigger inflammation, which can drive hormonal dysfunction. Likewise, hormonal imbalances disrupt the vaginal microbiome. For example, low oestrogen levels can lead to bacterial overgrowth in the vaginal microbiome, creating an inflammatory environment and triggering inflammation that could in turn exacerbate hormone imbalances in a vicious cycle. An imbalance increases your susceptibility to opportunistic bacteria, which in turn increases your risk of chronic infection, which can drive inflammation in the body.

An imbalance of vaginal flora has also been linked to infertility, unsuccessful embryo implantation, preterm birth, endometriosis, PCOS, recurring UTIs, thrush (yeast infections), bacterial vaginosis, vulvovaginal itching vaginal dryness, painful intercourse, increased risk of thrush, bacterial vaginosis, and urinary tract infections. It may increase your likelihood of contracting an STI if you are exposed.

An imbalanced vaginal microbiome in early pregnancy, particularly high levels of *Gardnerella vaginalis*, has been linked to an increased risk of miscarriage. This bacteria reduces *Lactobacillus* and disrupts the vaginal flora. Studies also show recurrent miscarriages are often associated with infections like bacterial vaginosis, fungal vaginosis, Group B streptococcus, or mycoplasma infection.

Low oestrogen states (e.g. perimenopause, menopause, PCOS, breastfeeding, oral contraceptives) can lead to vaginal dysbiosis, while high oestrogen states (e.g. endometriosis, oral contraceptives, or HRT) may protect the microbiome but increase the risk of fungal overgrowth.

HORMONES AND YOUR VAGINAL MICROBIOME

Your vaginal microbiome and hormones are deeply interconnected, each shaping the other continuously. The vaginal microbiome sees slight fluctuations in its composition during each phase of the menstrual cycle. Healthy oestrogen levels will support a healthy vaginal flora composition.

A balanced vaginal microbiome can prevent inflammation by protecting against bacterial overgrowth and potentially harmful microbes like strep B), maintaining overall vaginal health.

The vaginal microbiome also fluctuates during pregnancy, when nearly every organ system in the body changes and adapts to help promote a healthy pregnancy outcome. The preponderance of *Lactobacillus* in pregnancy appears to be aided by the oestrogen-induced increase in glycogen that contributes to the vaginal acidic environment. This is not only enhanced by *Lactobacilli*, but also fosters *Lactobacillus* growth, which can be protective.

Your Liver and Hormones

Fondly referred to as the body's "biochemical laboratory", the liver is a major player in your endocrine function. Recent research highlights the liver as a key organ in regulating metabolism.

Despite what some juice cleanses, supplements, and "detox" teas may have promised, nothing can "detox" your body besides your own organs. You can support the process of detoxification, but no product will do it for you.

THE LIVER'S ROLE

The liver performs many functions in the body, known as hepatic functions (see opposite). A number of these functions are key to the production and regulation of hormones. Half endocrine gland, half exocrine gland (see p.80 for more on the endocrine system), the liver does a lot.

Where hormones are concerned, the liver acts as the body's laboratory, producing (among other things) most of the cholesterol the body needs. Given that cholesterol is where so many of our hormones begin (see p.30), it's imperative that we keep this organ in tip-top condition for the sake of optimal hormonal function. It also regulates your sex hormones by metabolizing them and providing a transport system (like the sex hormone–binding globulins, which we discussed on p.82).

ENDOCRINE VS EXOCRINE GLAND

An endocrine gland is an organ that produces hormones that are released into the blood. An exocrine gland produces and releases substances through ducts or openings – like digestive juices, sweat, tears, saliva, and milk.

Finally, the liver detoxifies hormones. Along with the gut, it is responsible for eliminating excess hormones that are no longer needed, acting as a sophisticated filtration system that breaks down and removes hormones from the bloodstream. If the liver is not functioning optimally, it can lead to an accumulation of hormones and, therefore, imbalances.

This process includes testosterone, cortisol, and progesterone, but it is also critical for oestrogen. Strongly influenced by nutrition (see p.164), it is critical that we support oestrogen detoxification, as otherwise we run the risk of oestrogen dominance and even oestrogen-dominant cancers. A build up of oestrogen comes with serious health risks, and further risks if its transformation is not optimal. For your liver to detoxify hormones, it must change their structure. This allows them to be excreted by the liver, but there is potential for toxicity during this three-phase process.

HORMONAL HEPATIC FUNCTION:	NON-HORMONAL HEPATIC FUNCTION:
Cholesterol synthesis	Bile secretion to aid fat digestion
Hormone detoxification and clearance	Fat creation, including the synthesis of triglycerides (and cholesterol)
Hormone metabolism, including your thyroid hormones	Glucose production
Hormone production, like vitamin D and insulin-like growth factor 1 (IGF-1)	Storage and metabolism of nutrients, vitamins, and micronutrients
Network for your sex and steroid hormones	Synthesis and storage of glycogen
Synthesis and regulation of blood proteins, including their transportation	

THE THREE PHASES OF OESTROGEN DETOXIFICATION

Your sex hormones are fat-based (lipophilic), and therefore must be converted into a water-soluble form in order to be excreted via your urine and stool. This is what we call the biotransformation of a lipophilic compound to a water-soluble compound. In the liver, this biotransformation happens in three phases.

PHASE I

In this first phase, the liver modifies oestrogen into metabolites, using the CYP family of enzymes. So far, so simple – except there are a huge number of different CYP enzymes, all competing with one another and interacting with oestrogen in different ways, known as "pathways".

There are three pathways, but let's focus on the ideal one, known as Pathway 2, using CYP1A1. Unlike the other pathways, which can convert oestrogen into potentially more toxic intermediate metabolites, Pathway 2 creates the most stable metabolite, known as 2–OH. This metabolite won't stimulate cell growth, and can block the action of stronger oestrogens (which might otherwise cause hormone imbalances).

To promote this pathway, encourage the availability of the CYP1A1 enzyme – natural inducers of this enzyme are found in the cruciferous family, including broccoli, brussels sprouts, and cabbage. Phase I can be compromised by alcohol, excessive caffeine, smoking, vaping, or endocrine-disrupting chemicals.

PHASE II

After oestrogen gains an -OH group (hydroxylation), an additional conjugating substance increases water solubility. This is where the body prepares harmful byproducts from Phase I for safe removal, making the oestrogen metabolites less bioactive. It does this via six pathways.

PHASE III

Finally, oestrogen metabolites (along with other toxins and hormones) are prepared for excretion. If this biotransformation process gets out of rhythm, there can be a hormonal pile-up. Phase I, II, and III need to be running in sync, like a coordinated assembly line. If Phase I operates at a faster rate than Phase II, it can result in an accumulation of byproducts, comparable to an overflowing bathtub. Likewise, if Phase III is blocked and sluggish, hormones can get piled up, recirculating in the body and potentially driving hormonal imbalance. In other words, too much oestrogen can build up in the liver, eventually spilling out and re-entering your system. This can lead to damage to cell proteins RNA and DNA, not to mention putting you at risk of oestrogen excess.

Basically, the aim is to get both Phase I and Phase II synchronized and stable. Much of this comes down to the diet, as covered in the first three pillars of the Positive Method – although for a more targeted approach to stablizing each phase, there are a few particular micronutrients you should champion in your meals.

WHAT HELPS KEEP PHASE I STABLE?

Antioxidants (e.g. cysteine, glycine, glutamine)

Zinc

Magnesium

B vitamins

WHAT HELPS KEEP PHASE II STABLE?

Cruciferous vegetables (e.g. broccoli, cauliflower, cabbage, sprouts)

Antioxidants (e.g. cysteine, glycine, glutamine)

Curcumin (found in turmeric)

Green tea

Magnesium

Vitamin A

Choline

OESTROGEN AND CONSTIPATION

Maintain a stable Phase III by supporting regular bowel movements with high-fibre foods. Top Tip: if you suffer with irregular bowel movements, try eating two kiwis a day with the skin on.

DETOXIFICATION AND LIVER DISEASE

With increasing cases of non-alcoholic fatty liver disease, liver health is generally declining. This increase runs parallel with rising obesity and diabetes rates among countries that consume foods high in ultra-processed foods. These foods are linked to higher levels of insulin, which push the liver to store fat.

This pressure on your liver is concerning because it represents the final step in your hormone processing; if the hormone's journey is scuppered, there can be serious consequences. That's why it's so important to take steps to reduce your toxic load right from the start.

If your liver is busy processing and detoxifying toxins and endocrine disruptors, it will prioritize clearing these toxins over your hormones. Where there is a burden on the liver, it can become overwhelmed and won't optimally regulate and remove hormones. This can lead to hormonal imbalance.

During the detoxification process, free radicals are produced as a by-product. This is why it's so important to eat a colourful rainbow of foods – all those powerful antioxidants will help mop up the free radicals.

The Triple Threat to Hormonal Health

Hormone imbalance arises from genetic and environmental factors. Insulin resistance, stress, and inflammation are in the driving seat, alongside gut imbalances, nutrient deficiencies, an unstable circadian rhythm, and exposure to endocrine disruptors (see p.109).

The good news is that, with the right guidance, we can all make better decisions. Some factors may fall outside of your control, but positive decisions can still have a major impact.

THE THREE THREATS

There are three main drivers that can influence the four phases of hormone health: insulin resistance, chronic inflammation, and stress.

Using the six pillars of the Positive Method (see p.118), you can learn how to control these drivers. The Positive Method is based on improving your insulin sensitivity, reducing inflammation, and supporting healthy cortisol levels.

THREAT 1: INSULIN RESISTANCE

Insulin resistance occurs when your body begins to resist the help insulin is trying to provide. After years of a chronic and continuous need for insulin, whether to mop up sugary excess or store fat, more insulin is needed for the same job.

HOW INSULIN RESISTANCE HAPPENS

The more you rely on insulin to clear excess glucose, the closer you get to insulin resistance. This happens because your cells become less sensitive to insulin with prolonged exposure. Your body starts to resist it, much like how you may start to need more caffeine if you increase your daily espresso intake. The more frequent your sugar spikes, the less responsive your cells become to insulin. As your cells build a tolerance, insulin becomes less effective. Eventually, your pancreas may struggle to keep up with the demand, leading to the need for insulin injections to manage regular glucose spikes.

INSULIN RESISTANCE, DIABETES, AND YOUR HEALTH

The medical definition of type 2 diabetes (T2DM) is an impaired biologic response to insulin stimulation. Lifestyle plays a major role, although some people are genetically predisposed to it, making them more at risk. Additionally, your life stage can also be an important factor (see opposite).

Insulin resistance doesn't just make you a bit bad at dealing with glucose; it negatively impacts many pathways for your hormones and propels your body into fat storage mode. There are repercussions across the board for your health. Remember, though, that while diet and lifestyle can cause type 2 diabetes, they can also be the same tools that put this disease into remission. What you eat, how you move, and the environment you create can all help insulin do its job.

INSULIN RESISTANCE AND YOUR SEX HORMONES

Insulin resistance can negatively impact your sex hormone binding globulin (SHBG) levels, which means the transportation system for your sex hormones can become compromised, contributing to issues such as excess testosterone.

Excess androgens, like testosterone, can disrupt your oestrogen levels by interfering with your oestrogen receptors – your hormone docking stations. If the docking station is damaged, you can be sure that the message to be delivered will also be damaged. Testosterone can also reduce the production of oestradiol, a key form of oestrogen, by blocking oestrogen receptor alpha (ERα), which can affect the body's ability to convert testosterone to oestrogen.

The body has two types of oestrogen receptors: ERα and ERβ. These receptors help regulate key functions across various systems, including your reproductive, skeletal, cardiovascular, and central nervous systems, as well as tissues like your breasts and ovaries. This is how oestradiol communicates messages throughout the body, impacting your physiology and behaviour.

INSULIN RESISTANCE AND MENOPAUSE

As you age, you are at greater risk of insulin resistance due to the drop in your sex hormones, namely oestradiol. This can worsen any existing hormone dysfunction, and even further lower your oestrogen levels if insulin resistance persists.

Insulin sensitivity is integral to your hormone health. If you're reading this as a younger woman, implementing positive change now will significantly benefit your hormonal health and improve your experience of menopause.

As ageing increases the risk of insulin resistance, it also increases the risk of type 2 diabetes. One study analyzed the effect of menopause age on type 2 diabetes risk in postmenopausal women. It found that earlier menopause is linked to a higher risk of developing T2DM, with the risk rising as menopause occurs earlier. Another recent study found that premenopausal women exhibit enhanced insulin sensitivity and reduced incidence of type 2 diabetes compared with age-matched men. However, with disrupted glucose levels, this female advantage disappears after menopause, in part owing to a reduction in circulating oestradiol. This is not just about hormones, ladies – this is about longevity.

ISSUES ASSOCIATED WITH INSULIN RESISTANCE:

Metabolic syndrome, a collection of conditions that occur together, increasing your risk of heart disease, stroke, and type 2 diabetes

Prediabetes or type 2 diabetes, conditions affecting blood sugar levels

Non-alcoholic fatty liver disease (NAFLD), a condition where fat builds up in the liver

Polycystic ovarian syndrome (PCOS) via insulin resistance's ability to raise androgen levels

Obesity

Raised LDL cholesterol and triglycerides

Microvascular disease (retinopathy, neuropathy, or nephropathy), conditions that affect the small blood vessels in the heart, brain, or other organs

Macrovascular disease (stroke, peripheral artery disease, coronary artery disease), conditions that affect the body's large blood vessels, such as the coronary arteries, aorta, and arteries in the brain and limbs

High blood pressure

INSULIN AND OESTROGEN DEPLETION

High insulin comes with high testosterone and compromised oestrogen signalling and production.

With high levels of testosterone, your target receptors become blind to oestrogen. The hormone cannot deliver its message.

Why is this a problem? If lacking in oestradiol, the large number of oestrogen cell receptors – from your brain to your breasts, vagina, skin, liver, and immune cells – will no longer be able to function optimally. If your brain is depleted of oestrogen, your entire organ system will have trouble functioning.

RISING INSULIN AND OESTROGEN

Frustratingly, what can also happen through a negative loop system is that the body thinks there is less oestrogen in circulation, so starts pumping more testosterone into your system – this is because, as we've learned, oestrogen is created from testosterone. This can spark a vicious cycle.

Oestrogen is indirectly affected by insulin resistance due to rising testosterone levels. However, it also improves insulin sensitivity by helping cells respond more effectively to insulin.

INSULIN RESISTANCE AND ENDOCRINE DISORDERS

Insulin resistance is a major factor in endocrine disorders like PCOS, which is driven by excess androgens.

Insulin can stimulate ovarian androgen production in normal women and women with PCOS. Insulin resistance also plays a complex but undeniable role in the transportation of your sex hormones, as insulin resistance can impact your sex hormone binding globulins (SHBG). Research conducted in the mid-1990s by the Endocrine Society has shown that insulin levels can decrease circulating SHBG, and suggests a close metabolic link between SHBG and insulin. Insulin resistance has also been found across longitudinal and cross-sectional studies in 2019 research. All this indicates that, as insulin resistance increases, SHBG levels are likely to decrease. This is going to lead to a rather long backlog of "free" unbound sex hormones in the bloodstream, as your

SHBGs can't efficiently transport your hormones to their target cells. This can drive up an excess of "free" testosterone in the system which, as you know, can manifest in a number of ways.

TESTING FOR INSULIN RESISTANCE

How do you know if you have insulin resistance? It can be tricky to diagnose, which is why it is so important to listen to your body and consider your existing risk factors (your age, or a family history of diabetes or insulin resistance). Insulin resistance is diagnosed by tests such as the fasting plasma glucose test (FBG), HbA1C test, or oral glucose tolerance test.

An HbA1C test captures your average blood sugar levels over three months. However, it is not very sensitive, and prediabetes can still be missed. A fasting plasma glucose test and oral glucose tolerance test both offer a time stamp of the amount of sugar in your blood at the specific time of the test. Examples of time-specific readings include:

HbAIC – 5.7 to 6.4 per cent sugar in your blood
FPG – 100 to 125 mg/dL (milligrams per decilitre)

Insulin sensitivity and insulin resistance operate on a broad spectrum. Just as there are different levels of physical fitness and strength, there are varying degrees as to how effectively your body manages glucose. Insulin resistance develops gradually, with glucose control worsening in stages. A decline in glucose management might not be immediately visible within blood tests, creating a grey area where issues could go undetected.

PHYSICAL SIGNS THAT COULD INDICATE INSULIN RESISTANCE:

Acanthosis nigricans – dark, thick, velvety skin around the neck, armpits, or groin, prevalent in individuals with PCOS

Skin tags

A waist to height ratio of over 0.5

OTHER SYMPTOMS I LOOK OUT FOR IN CLINIC:

Sweet cravings, particularly at 11 am, 3 pm, and 9 pm

Refined carbohydrate cravings

Low energy

Brain fog

Midday fatigue or after eating

Hunger shortly after eating

Irritability

Headaches

INSULIN RESISTANCE AND INFLAMMATION

Finally, where there is insulin resistance, there will be inflammation. Inflammation is a smart defensive system that recognizes potential dangers to your immunity and eliminates harmful stimuli in your body. It does this so that you can then repair and heal, and forms a core part of your immune system. However, anything in excess can be dangerous for the body, and chronic inflammation is no different.

Insulin resistance and inflammation have a reciprocal relationship that can lead to deteriorating metabolic dysfunction. They operate in a vicious cycle – insulin resistance can result in more inflammation, and more inflammation can drive more insulin resistance. This dynamic makes managing insulin resistance even more challenging, and can create a hostile environment for your hormone balance and overall health.

THREAT 2: STRESS

As we have already learned (see pp.56–63), fear or stress can trigger elevated cortisol and adrenaline levels as part of our "fight-or-flight" instincts. When you find yourself in this nervous state, your body limits all other non-essential functions, which could include anything from your reproductive function to your digestion. Your body is hardwired to survive, and this core biological drive will override everything else. The problem comes when your body is being constantly burdened, on a chronic level, by this drive to survive.

CORTISOL CRISIS

From Gen Alpha to Z, millennials to boomers, there is no doubt that we are living in an age of cortisol crisis. So many individuals are experiencing chronic levels of stress because of the sheer number of stimuli we face. As we become less adept at switching off, this list grows longer.

Any physical or psychological stimuli, real or perceived, can disrupt your biological homeostasis and result in a stress response. It is one of the biggest roadblocks that I see in my private clinic. However, with the right support tools, it can be addressed – with life-changing positive results.

HIGH CORTISOL SYMPTOMS:

Anxiety	Low progesterone levels
Compromised sleep	Memory loss
Depression	Recurring illness
Elevated androgens	Stubborn abdominal fat
Hair loss	Thyroid dysfunction
Irritability	

STRESS AND DIET

Research has shown that stress influences our eating behaviour. Not only that, but what we eat can in turn escalate cortisol levels – caffeine, alcohol, saturated fat, sugar, and ultra-processed foods all play their part. This leads to a vicious circle of high cortisol leading to poor food choices, and poor food choices leading to high cortisol. Research has concluded that obesity is being driven in part by the preponderance of chronic stress, as elevated cortisol can promote the desire to seek high-fat, energy-dense foods. When cortisol negatively impacts your food intake by leading you towards ultra-processed foods, it can drive nutrient deficiency and inflammation – a tough environment for your hormones to thrive in.

THE SYMPATHETIC NERVOUS SYSTEM (SNS)

The sympathetic nervous system (SNS) controls the "fight-or-flight" response, activated during stress, danger, or physical activity. It increases heart rate, blood pressure, and sweating, while slowing digestion.

The parasympathetic nervous system (PNS), on the other hand, is responsible for the "rest and digest" state. It calms the body after stress, slowing the heart rate and restarting digestion, eventually restoring balance after the SNS response.

COUNTERACTING STRESS

When stress levels are consistently high, cortisol can override your endocrine system. In practical terms, this can lead to issues such as weight gain, facial puffiness, poor sleep, lack of appetite in the morning, irritability, and changes to your sex drive – clear signs that the body is out of balance. This makes it harder for your other hormones to communicate and causes chaos. Although cortisol is setting out to help you, its impact, when elevated, can be dramatic, ultimately turning up the volume on insulin resistance.

Changing the narrative for your nervous system is crucial to remind yourself that you are not in danger. Take time each day to bring yourself into the present. Activities like slowing down, swapping high-intensity workouts for yoga, practising breathwork, and spending time outdoors can help calm the nervous system. We'll explore this more in Pillar Five (see p.184).

STRESS, CORTISOL, AND INSULIN

Cortisol can also encourage insulin resistance, ensuring there is energy at hand – an evolutionary tool in a "fight-or-flight" scenario, but less helpful to us nowadays. If your body is out to ensure your survival, cortisol is damn sure to keep any energy-rich substrate like glucose readily available. As a result, cortisol will block the energy storage into your muscles, liver, and fat tissue by interfering with insulin – it dials up the mechanism of insulin resistance that stops you from storing glucose as energy. Cortisol has the ability to create energy for you, as when you are stressed your body can create glucose via the liver for energy.

Insulin functions like a lock and key, unlocking space in your body to store glucose molecules in order to move them out of your bloodstream. Elevated cortisol jams up the system, increasing the demand for insulin to manage blood sugar, putting pressure on your system to create more insulin, and potentially driving insulin resistance.

THREAT 3: DIET-INDUCED INFLAMMATION

Where we have a high level of excess circulating cortisol, there will be inflammation. And, as you now know, where we have insulin resistance, there will be inflammation. Excess androgens are strongly associated with chronic inflammation, as is eating a diet comprised largely of ultra-processed foods. Inflammation is linked with an excess of body fat, while obesity itself can trigger an inflammatory state in metabolic tissues. This is because fat cells actually act as an endocrine organ, producing both hormones and inflammatory cytokines (see p.108).

In other words, inflammation has a huge number of causes – and, when experienced on a chronic level, it can compromise not only your hormonal health but general health too. It manifests as pain and immune dysfunction, and can damage healthy cells, tissues, and organs, leading to disease.

Where there is inflammation, there may also be a compromised gut – and a compromised gut will disrupt your hormones (see Pillar Two, p.137). Inflammation can be acute or it can be chronic. In this case, we are talking about the latter, which is slow, steady, and constant inflammation.

TESTING FOR INFLAMMATION

When you are looking out for inflammation through blood tests, you're normally on the hunt for elevated serum levels of C-reactive protein (CRP). This is a protein that is made by your liver in response to inflammation via the release of interleukin-6 (IL-6), which is a type of cytokine that is

CYTOKINES

Cytokines are small proteins that act as messengers for the immune system, alerting it to threats like pathogens and antigens. Like a defence team, they coordinate immune cell responses to infections and regulate the growth and activity of immune and blood cells, playing a key role in both acute and chronic inflammation.

secreted to promote inflammation. The presence of this protein can be a good marker for chronic inflammation – but this isn't always the case. You most definitely can suffer from chronic inflammation, even if this marker is not notably raised.

In the throes of stage 4 endometriosis, I was someone who did not demonstrate elevated levels of C-reactive protein. I was turned away multiple times by a GP, who told me I could not have endometriosis. They were incorrect. If ever there was a condition linked to inflammation, endometriosis is it!

When it comes to endocrine disorders, much of the literature links chronic inflammation as a principal driver, although we need to understand more of the mechanics. The exact mechanism of inflammation in endometriosis and PCOS still remains largely unknown, but we do know the link is there.

The Four Ps of Hormone Disruption

So, we've learnt about a number of key hormones, as well as key bodily systems and the main threats to hormone health. Before we dive into the Positive Method and take steps to rebalancing our hormones, it's worth taking a moment to look at four lifestyle factors that can really cause disruption. Let's meet the four Ps:

PLASTICS
PRODUCTS
PESTICIDES
PEOPLE

Toxins are everywhere these days, from your makeup bag to your cleaning arsenal. In fact, your home plays host to a whole cocktail of hormone-disrupting chemicals. It's vital to take some time now for a bit of a clear-out, decluttering and making some healthier swaps in your living space.

In chapter 1, we looked at how the landscape of hormones has changed over the years thanks to the impact of forever chemicals, plastics, and the fast-paced modern world we live in. Understanding these changes helps to identify the practical steps you can take in reducing your exposure to endocrine-disrupting chemicals.

ENDOCRINE DISRUPTORS

The term "endocrine disruptor" refers to any chemical compound that can significantly affect your endocrine system (see pp.80–83). They do this by mimicking your hormones, blocking your cell receptors so that those all-important messages can't be delivered, influencing your hormone production and interfering with hormone signalling.

Endocrine disruptors can be artificially made or naturally occurring, disrupting your hormones and interfering with the regular functioning of your endocrine system, not to mention your reproductive system and any other biological processes that your hormones regulate.

This can have serious implications for everyone, but especially developing foetuses and infants or those going through hormonal changes during puberty, as well as women with PCOS, other endocrine disorders, or entering into perimenopause. Addressing the four Ps – plastics, products, pesticides, and people – offers another way of turning down the volume on your symptoms. Let's look at how to reduce them.

FOREIGN OESTROGENS

Special attention should be given to a group known as xenoestrogens – otherwise known as "foreign oestrogens". These synthetic chemicals include certain medications, pesticides, and industrial byproducts that can disrupt regular oestrogen signalling by binding to oestrogen receptors and even mimicking oestrogen by demonstrating oestrogen-like activity. Their negative impact may be heightened if your oestrogen levels are low or decreasing as during perimenopause, as there will be more empty oestrogen receptors ready to latch onto these troublesome chemicals.

Phytoestrogens also technically fall into this foreign oestrogen category. Unlike synthetic xenoestrogens, though, phytoestrogens are derived from plants – think soybeans, edamame, flaxseed, apples, pears, beans, sprouts, cabbage, and spinach. We can use phytoestrogens to our advantage because they have a whole host of oestrogen balancing benefits. We'll talk more about this in Pillar Two (see p.137).

FOREVER CHEMICALS

You may question whether so-called "forever chemicals" can cross the skin barrier. Named for their resistance to breakdown, these substances remain in the environment (and potentially in your body) for a very long time. The skin, made of dense layers like the epidermis, is designed to protect against toxins and pathogens. The outer layer, the stratum corneum, is packed with lipids, keratin, and dead skin cells, acting as the body's first line of defence.

CHEMICALS THAT MIGHT INTERFERE WITH THE HORMONES:*

PESTICIDES

Chemicals like atrazine
and organophosphate
commonly found
in non-organic foods.

PHTHALATES

Present in nail polish,
shampoos, conditioners, and
many cosmetics that list
"fragrance" as an ingredient.

PARABENS

Used in shampoos, conditioners,
cosmetics, and sanitary items.

HEAVY METALS

Such as lead, which can be
found in paint, toys, and plumbing,
and mercury, which is often
present in seafood.

PFAS

Found in non-stick cookware,
water-resistant clothing, tap water,
and stain-resistant furniture.

CHEMICAL UV FILTERS

Certain ingredients
used in sunscreens,
like oxybenzone.

BPA AND BPA ALTERNATIVES

Commonly found in plastic
food and drink packaging,
the linings of tin cans, thermal
paper receipts, and water bottles.

ALUMINIUM (ALUMINUM)

Found in cookware,
food packaging,
antiperspirants,
and drinking water.

*chemicals include, but are not limited to, this list

However, some harmful chemicals, like PFAS, can penetrate this barrier. A 2024 study from the University of Birmingham confirmed that 15 out of 17 PFAS tested were absorbed through the skin, with 13.5 per cent of perfluorooctanoic acid (PFOA) entering the bloodstream.

The skin barrier's effectiveness can be weakened by factors such as sun exposure, harsh weather, dry or humid environments, pollution, allergens, and over-washing. Even products like strong soaps and retinol can damage it, increasing the risk of toxin absorption.

Additionally, chemicals can enter your body through hand-to-mouth contact or by ingesting residues from surfaces – lipsticks, for instance, have been shown to contain heavy metals, with one study estimating the metal intake for average lipstick users as 24 mg (0.00085 oz) a day, and high lipstick users 87 mg (0.003 oz) per day. Those numbers soon add up!

SANITARY PRODUCTS

Sanitary products have recently come under the spotlight following a systematic review that investigated the chemicals found in these items. Anything applied directly to your skin or in your mouth is going to be readily absorbed, but your vaginal and vulvar tissues are particularly sensitive and highly permeable – chemicals absorbed here can enter the bloodstream without going through first-pass metabolism. Shockingly, the study on sanitary products actually detected phthalates, volatile organic compounds, parabens, environmental phenols, fragrance chemicals, dioxins, and dioxin-like compounds in a number of menstrual products, concluding that "[...] menstrual products contained measurable levels of a range of endocrine-disrupting chemicals including phthalates, phenols, and parabens". This is particularly alarming when you think of the average menstruating woman, who will use over 11,000 tampons or sanitary pads in their lifetime. The combination of high absorption rates in this sensitive area and prolonged exposure over time is a serious concern.

PEOPLE

Now, I know that people don't contain chemicals that disrupt hormones, but some people and relationships can be tricky. By reducing the time you spend with energy vampires – people who are demanding, toxic, or make you feel bad about yourself – you'll create a happier home for your hormones. We'll talk more about this in Pillar Six (see p.195).

EASY SWAPS

The quest for cleaner living can feel daunting and sometimes near impossible, but there are always opportunities to make some simple changes. Remember that it's about *limiting*, not eliminating. Putting too much pressure on yourself to live a completely non-toxic life will become overwhelming fast, and the truth is, you can't get away from every single one of these chemicals, as many are just now a part of our world.

I have made some major swaps in my kitchen, fridge, and make-up bag over the years, but you won't see me getting ride of my Diptyque perfume or Dior mascara anytime soon. On the other hand, I've happily parted ways with things like plastic food containers, non-stick pans, toxic sanitary products, plastic chopping boards, cling film, toxic surface cleaners, standard dishwasher tablets, certain sunscreens, unfiltered tap water, and deodorant containing aluminium (aluminum). Still, some things remain – and they can for you, too.

DECIPHERING LABELS
I'm going to share a secret weapon that I've used for years! There are some excellent apps where you can search and scan products to see how toxic they are. It's a great tool if you struggle understanding labels.

YOUR LIFE PANTRY CLEAR-OUT SWAPS:
Let's set the scene: today is day one of your home clear-out. Identify where you can make swaps – what is going to best suit your current home set-up? Where could you make better decisions with plastics, products, pesticides, and people? Pull up your sleeves; it's time to clear out as much toxic energy as possible before we start Pillar One.

Sanitary products	→	Non-toxic organic sanitary towels (pads) or menstrual cup
Plastic chopping board	→	Wooden chopping board
Cling film (plastic wrap)	→	Beeswax covers or saucers to cover food
Foil	→	Parchment paper
Plastic bottles	→	Stainless-steel or glass water bottles
Plastic storage boxes	→	Glass or stainless-steel containers
Plastic-wrapped snacks	→	Stainless-steel lunch boxes
Non-stick cookware	→	Stainless-steel or non-toxic pans

… And a final, easy one: leave your shoes by the front door to avoid tracking in any unwanted substances!

Remember to pick your battles! By getting some of the above swaps in, you'll have made a sterling start to creating a happier environment for your hormones in your home.

THE FINAL "P": PERSPECTIVE

Endocrine disruptors come in various forms, and it's important to identify the main sources to limit your exposure. As much as we might want to, we can't change everything about our lives. Switching every plastic item in our home for a wooden equivalent might be too costly to do all at once, while finding organic swaps for all our favourite foods can take time. The best thing we can do is pick our battles and make changes wherever we can.

One issue I do recommend making an immediate switch on, if you're using them, is sanitary products, for the reasons listed above. Make an easy swap to a reputable organic brand, or try using a menstrual cup. The jury may still be out on sanitary underwear, so be sure to always do your research.

I am a realist. As a working mum, there are times when I need a stronger cleaning product, and I'm not looking to make life any harder when it comes to keeping the house in order. Small changes can make a difference. I also love my beauty products and anti-wrinkle serums, but I make sure to research the ingredients – and you should too.

When it comes to "clean" cleaning products, a huge variety of brands have hit the shelves, from eco-friendly dishwasher sheets to surface sprays made with essential oils. There are also the more traditional cleaning methods that use white wine vinegar, bicarbonate of soda (baking soda), lemon juice, and a bit of elbow grease. It's not just what you eat – our environment matters just as much.

There are times when only bleach or a bit of stain remover will do. But if you can reduce your everyday use of toxic products, you'll reduce the cumulative effect of these harmful chemicals. As with ultra-processed food, occasional exposure to chemicals is unlikely to drive dramatic hormone disruption, in the same way that one ultra-processed chocolate bar is not going to undo a fabulous week of whole foods. You can't avoid ultra-processed foods completely, and it's even harder to avoid endocrine-disrupting hormones. What matters is what you do the majority of the time. As with nutrition, this is not about perfection, but about doing the best that you can.

3.

The
Positive
Method

The Six Pillars

PILLAR ONE
HEY SUGAR,
LET'S BALANCE
P. 125

PILLAR TWO
EAT
COLOURFUL
P. 137

PILLAR THREE
EAT SMART
P. 159

PILLAR FOUR
MOVE MORE
P. 174

PILLAR FIVE
SLEEP BETTER
P. 184

PILLAR SIX
LIVE POSITIVE
P. 195

Taking Positive Action

Let's begin implementing positive actions to support your body and work in harmony with your hormones. You'll be guided by Six Pillars, filled with actionable steps you can apply to your own life. I call this the Positive Method, an evidence-based approach combining the knowledge you have gained about hormonal health with actionable tools and steps to create a happier home for your hormones.

This programme addresses both nutrition and the "triple threat" of hormonal imbalance – insulin sensitivity, inflammation, and stress. It also focuses on sleep, muscle mass, and the gut and vaginal microbiome. Throughout, emotional wellbeing is central. After all, every aspect of your life – from the food you eat to the people you surround yourself with, your daily movement, bedtime, and mental health – affects your hormonal balance.

Hormonal symptoms are signals from your body indicating something deeper is going on. To truly resolve these imbalances, you need to look at the root cause. The Positive Method is not just about an individual food, trendy supplement, or exercise regime. It's a holistic, multifaceted approach to address the root causes of hormonal dysfunction by positively impacting the four stages of hormone health.

It also isn't a quick fix. Imagine this journey like a beautiful tapestry, unique to you. This is an opportunity to create lasting change for the rest of your life. While results might come quickly, remember to go at your own pace. I recommend introducing one pillar every two weeks.

The method will be something you can return to anytime you need it. As you continue, you'll introduce new tools, strategies, and small but positive clinically backed changes. Take your time, trust the process, and allow your transformation to unfold at its own pace.

GETTING STARTED

First, let's take a moment to reflect on where you are right now. You have probably picked up this book because you suspect you're experiencing hormonal dysfunction, whether that's because you've noticed certain symptoms, or because you have received (or are seeking) a diagnosis for a hormone-related issue.

HAVE YOU NOTICED RECURRING ISSUES AROUND

Fatigue, low energy, poor sleep, or insomnia

Irregular, heavy, or painful periods or infertility

Fluctuations in weight

Bloating, constipation, or digestion

Mood swings, irritability, anxiety, or brain fog

Hair loss, acne, or other skin problems

YOU MAY HAVE BEEN DIAGNOSED WITH

PMS

PMDD

PCOS

Endometriosis

An underactive thyroid

Alternatively, you may be riding a hormonal shift and looking for ways to support your body through it. Navigating perimenopause, for example, is going to feel a lot more challenging and chaotic if your body is dealing with insulin resistance, inflammation and stress – symptoms that often arise during menopause.

NATURAL HORMONAL SHIFTS YOU COULD BE EXPERIENCING

Puberty

Pregnancy / Postnatal

Perimenopause / Menopause

It's also possible that you're experiencing a combination – a double whammy of a dysfunction accompanied by the challenges of a natural shift. The Positive Method is designed to support both hormonal shifts and dysfunction alike. The key to working in harmony with your hormones is giving them the chance to thrive.

SUPPORTING HORMONE FUNCTION

The main goal of the Positive Method is to encourage a healthy and happy endocrine system – the four-step process of hormone function (see pp.80–83). The Method is designed to teach you how best to eat, move, and sleep for hormonal balance, using a positive mindset and a flexible framework. You wont't find any strict meal schedules founded on restriction. Instead, I've developed a "styling" formula for food, as well as lifestyle adjustments and tools to reduce stress by fostering happiness and positive actions.

We'll take it step by step. The power is in your hands.

SETTING YOUR SUCCESS STORY

Before we dive into each pillar, let's get clear on your "why" – your reason for wanting to take charge of your hormonal health. This is the first step I take with my clients – now it's your turn. Grab a notebook and pen, and write down what has brought you to this point, and what you want to achieve as a result of following the Method. I have included some ideas opposite, but your "why" should be completely personal to you.

Write down:

....

Your success story

....

Your goals for the upcoming months

....

Your mantra

....

Defining your "why" is a crucial part of your journey, and an incredibly powerful tool. Whether you write it down or speak it out loud to help make it real, you are much more likely to stick to the Method and make long-lasting changes if you are clear about your motivation – and, by following the plan, you will be able to turn your "why" into your success story. In the weeks ahead, you'll be making some changes – changes that require commitment, and sometimes discipline.

When making new decisions about food or daily routines, having a clear "why" will keep you on track. On days when you don't feel like prepping your breakfast or lacing up your trainers (athletic shoes), remember why you're here and why you're doing this.

This journey is about positive change, not added stress. As with any major project, this journey requires preparation, planning, and purpose. You wouldn't dive into a big task without meetings, strategy, or support – and the same applies to your personal goals. Setting clear goals and creating a vision board is essential to defining success.

WHAT ARE YOUR AIMS? SOME RECENT CLIENT GOALS HAVE INCLUDED:

GENERAL WELLBEING
Feeling healthier, happier, less bloated, and at peace with food.

OVERALL HAPPINESS
Fostering a sense of calm, health, and happiness, living life fully.

WEIGHT MANAGEMENT
Getting to and maintaining a healthy weight, developing new habits while breaking old unhealthy ones.

PHYSICAL HEALTH
Improving skin health, normalizing menstrual cycles, alleviating headaches and gut symptoms, supporting joint flexibility.

HORMONAL AND REPRODUCTIVE HEALTH
Finding the root cause of PCOS, preparing for pregnancy, and managing symptoms related to menopause.

MENTAL AND EMOTIONAL HEALTH
Finding new ways to manage stress and anxiety, improve sleep, feel rested and energetic.

PRIORITIZING YOU

Remember, you're here for you. Many women I work with put themselves last, but now it's your turn to shine. By prioritizing you and becoming your best self, you can bring greater happiness, health, and joy to everyone around you.

What you imagine, you create. Your story isn't set in stone – it grows and changes with you, guiding you forward every step of the way.

It's never too late to change direction and become who you want to be.

TIME FOR A RESET

To support this goal-setting, let's begin with a physical reset of your living space. Perhaps you've already started making the hormone-friendly changes listed in the four Ps section on p.109.

RESTOCK

Start by reworking your weekly shopping list, removing any foods that don't support your goals. Whether it's chocolate or ultra-processed snacks, it's time to let them go.

Remember, your success is much more important than these quick fixes. While treats like crisps (chips), chocolate, and wine can fit into the Positive Method, minimizing access to the foods that don't align with your "why" will make the journey easier – especially at the start. If it's not in your home, you won't be tempted to reach for it.

DECLUTTER

Streamline your kitchen, bedroom, and mental space. Invest in some glass food containers and a stainless-steel water bottle. Delete any apps that negatively increase your screen time and drag you down emotionally. Treat yourself to some new activewear so that you feel motivated to move more when we come to Pillar Four (p.174). Set aside a notebook geared towards positivity – getting things down on paper will help remind you why you're on this journey.

Pillar One
Hey Sugar, Let's Balance

It's time to boost your energy, mental clarity and hormone balance by improving your insulin sensitivity. The goal here is simple: to prevent excess glucose from flooding your bloodstream by making smarter carbohydrate choices, reducing sugar intake, and timing your meals to maintain stable blood sugar. This will help enhance your body's sensitivity to insulin when it's needed – essentially giving your insulin a fitness boost.

We're going to create a simple framework for making easy meals that nourish your body without relying on restrictive measures like calorie counting.

UNDERSTANDING MACRONUTRIENTS

Balancing macronutrients is key to hormone health. These are the three essential building blocks of your diet: carbohydrates, fats, and protein. Your body can't produce these on its own, which is why they're considered essential.

In this pillar, we'll mostly be talking about carbohydrates, as these directly impact your blood sugar and insulin levels. However, it's worth understanding the vital role played by fats and proteins too, and how they can support a smoother ride for your glucose levels when paired with carbohydrates.

Macronutrient classification isn't black and white. Foods like nuts, seeds, and yoghurt can contain both protein and fat, while quinoa and beans are both carbs and protein. Almost all foods, except oil and vinegar, contain some protein. However, grouping foods can help you better manage glucose levels and identify the best sources of each macronutrient.

FATS

Fats are vital for your body. They are essential for producing your steroid and sex hormones, maintaining healthy cell structures and skin, storing energy, and absorbing fat-soluble vitamins like A, D, E, and K. Fats also help regulate your body temperature.

125

There are four main types of dietary fats: polyunsaturated fats (found in oily fish, vegetable oils, nuts, and seeds); monounsaturated fats (found in olive oil, avocados, and nuts); saturated fats (in animal products and coconut oil, some label this "bad", but current research suggests dietary cholesterol has a minimal impact on blood cholesterol and CVD risk); and trans fats (found in processed foods like margarine, which raise LDL cholesterol and increase risks of heart disease, stroke, and diabetes).

PROTEINS

Proteins are the body's building blocks, made up of amino acids linked by peptide bonds. There are about 20 different amino acids used in the body, nine of which are essential and must come from our diet.

Proteins are essential for repairing and rebuilding tissues and muscles, and for synthesising enzymes. They play a crucial role in producing hormones, antibodies, cytokines, and neurotransmitters. They transport hormones around the body, with the liver producing a number of different proteins, including SHBG, which bind and transport sex hormones, and albumin, the most abundant protein in blood plasma, which also transports hormones including cortisol and testosterone.

A common misconception is that protein is only found in animal-derived foods, including meat, fish, eggs, and dairy. There are also many plant-based foods rich in protein, such as nuts, seeds, legumes, wholegrains, tofu, and tempeh.

CARBOHYDRATES

Carbohydrates, your primary energy source, fuel your movement, nervous system and brain, while supporting hormone, gut and immune health. They include fibre (non-digestible) and simple sugars.

Carbohydrates play a pivotal role in regulating blood sugar levels, stimulating insulin release and determining how the body reserves energy by converting it into glycogen. Many carbohydrates are **starches**, which are long chains of glucose, providing energy. Found in foods such as potatoes, rice, and bread, they provide a steady source of energy to keep you fuelled throughout the day. However, not all carbohydrates are starches – think broccoli or honey.

SIMPLE CARBOHYDRATES

Simple carbohydrates consist of one or two sugar units, called monosaccharides and disaccharides. Because of their simple chemical structure, the body breaks them down quickly, causing a rapid rise in blood glucose levels. Common examples of these sugars include glucose, fructose, galactose, ribose, lactose, maltose, and sucrose.

Simple carbohydrates are found in chocolate, sweets, carbonated drinks, fruit juices, honey, table sugar, and maple syrup. These are known as refined simple carbohydrates, as the original structure has been stripped down and refined to artificially boost taste, texture, and addictiveness, minimizing the number of bonds. This includes refined grains devoid of bran and fibre like soft white bread, many breakfast cereals, white rice and pizza, pasta, or pastries made with white flour.

COMPLEX CARBOHYDRATES

Complex carbohydrates are made up of three or more sugar units, known as oligosaccharides or polysaccharides, linked in a more intricate structure. The greater the number of bonds, the longer these carbohydrates take to digest. This results in a slower, more gradual release of glucose into the bloodstream, avoiding those rapid spikes associated with simple carbohydrates. Examples of complex carbohydrates include cellulose, dextrin, and amylose.

This group includes many non-starchy vegetables, which add fibre and nutrients without rapidly raising blood sugar.

EXAMPLES INCLUDE:

Artichokes	Cabbage
Asparagus	Cauliflower
Bean sprouts	Celery
Broccoli	Cucumber

Green leafy vegetables	Peppers
Mushrooms	Spinach
Onions	Tomatoes

Starchy complex carbohydrates are the most structurally complex and contain the highest number of glucose molecule bonds. You will learn to incorporate and style these in your meals.

EXAMPLES INCLUDE, BUT ARE NOT LIMITED TO:

Wholegrains e.g. brown rice and quinoa	Starchy vegetables e.g. potatoes, legumes, peas, squash, and parsnips
Wheat products e.g. sourdough bread	

RESISTANT STARCH

Another essential type of carbohydrate is resistant starch. This occurs naturally in some foods, and can also be formed through certain cooking and cooling processes. True to its name, it "resists" digestion in the small intestine, and instead is fermented in the large intestine. There, it acts as a prebiotic (a type of food that promotes the growth of healthy bacteria), nourishing all of your lovely gut microbes.

Resistant starch bypasses standard digestion without converting to glucose molecules like other carbohydrates. It therefore leads to lower glucose entry into your bloodstream, and sometimes even none at all – excellent news for stabilizing blood sugar levels.

Cooling foods after cooking can increase resistant starch formation. For example, cooking a potato opens up its starch granules, making them more accessible to digestive enzymes. However, when the potato is cooled, the granules close up again, making them resistant to digestion.

IS SUGAR A SUGAR?

All sugar – white, brown, agave, or honey – will impact your blood sugar. It comes down to precisely the same glucose molecule. Even though two molecules might look the same at surface level, their composition makes all the difference. For example, while both raw honey and processed honey are forms of sugar, raw honey, has antibacterial properties and retains nutrients such as enzymes, antioxidants, and trace minerals, which processed honey loses during refinement. This is why raw honey on yogurt can offer more nutritional benefits than its processed counterpart as it can act as a prebiotic and stimulate the growth of friendly bacteria like *Lactobacillus* and *Bifidobacteria*.

The chemical structure of sugar can differ – whether naturally found alongside fibre, whether eaten in excessive amounts, whether it is a single-molecule monosaccharide or a two-unit disaccharide (see p.127). If sugar has been mindlessly added during food processing, its delivery into your system has the potential to be pro-inflammatory. Choosing a sugar with more nutritional benefits is always the smarter choice. Fruit, which also contains fibre, will cause less intense glucose spikes. Processing removes beneficial vitamins and minerals, so the less processed the sugar the better. If both sugar options have the potential to spike your glucose levels, you might as well go for the one with added nutritional benefits. Minimizing added sugar is a positive goal when seeking hormone balance. But don't let this demonize all sugars. Do not be afraid of a little honey or a few dried apricots. Dates have a high sugar content, but research shows that they are nutritionally beneficial, particularly regarding glycaemic control among patients with diabetes.

EXAMPLES INCLUDE:

Green bananas

Cooked and cooled potatoes, rice, and pasta

Legumes such as beans, lentils, and peas

Wholegrains like oats and barley

Plantains

FIBRE

Finally, we have fibre, a unique carbohydrate that is not digestible. It cannot be broken down or absorbed in the small intestine, and therefore does not affect your blood sugar levels – no glucose is released. Fibre is therefore an excellent addition for supporting balanced blood sugar.

EXAMPLES INCLUDE:

Fruits and vegetables

Wholegrains

Legumes

Nuts and seeds

Although fibre is technically a complex carbohydrate, its resistance to digestion allows it to act as fuel for beneficial gut bacteria, promoting healthy bacterial growth in the colon. Fibre also serves as a bulking agent, helping to keep your bowel movements regular. You will learn more about upping your fibre intake in Pillar Two on p.137.

THE DIGESTION PROCESS

When you eat, your body breaks food down into tiny pieces, allowing it to extract energy, primarily from carbohydrates. Starch is broken down into glucose, which is then converted into ATP – adenosine triphosphate, the body's preferred energy source. Depending on your body's needs, some of this energy is used immediately while the rest is stored.

Before glucose is converted into energy, it enters your bloodstream. The more complex the carbohydrate, the more bonds to break and the harder it is for your body to break it down. It's like cutting though 20 stacked pieces of rope instead of two – it takes more time and more effort. This slows the rate at which glucose enters your bloodstream.

Complex carbohydrates therefore have what's known as a low GI, or glycaemic (glycemic) index. GI measures the extent and speed at which a food raises blood sugar levels – the lower, the better.

At the opposite end of the scale, simple carbohydrates break down faster, causing a bigger, quicker spike in glucose levels. In other words, they are high GI foods.

Foods with a high GI will lead to a blood sugar crash, accompanied by low energy, increased hunger, and sugar cravings. You can see this with white bread, for example. When you're next in the company of white bread, take a small bite and chew it slowly, without swallowing. After about a minute, you begin to taste the sweetness. This is how quickly your saliva, aided by salivary amylase, breaks it down. Eating toasted white bread for breakfast will leave you feeling hungrier faster, with a more pronounced dip in your energy levels. Opting instead for a slice of toasted dark rye bread, which is more nutritionally complex and, thanks to its high soluble fibre content, has a lower GI, will provide more material for your digestion to break down and slow the rate at which glucose enters your bloodstream. Eating rye bread will lead to a more gradual rise in your blood sugar levels than white bread, meaning you'll feel fuller for longer and can avoid a crash.

If too much glucose enters into your bloodstream at once, it can lead to problems. Excessive glucose is inflammatory. It's also extremely sticky (think of the stickiness of caramel!) and puts enormous strain on your arteries. This is what's known as a glucose spike. It's normal to encounter these, but frequent spikes can harm your health.

THE BLOOD SUGAR ROLLER COASTER

It's not just high GI foods that can cause a spike. They can also occur when we eat too much sugar, excess carbohydrates, or "naked carbs" – carbohydrates eaten alone without fat and protein. Your ability to metabolize glucose can also be influenced by genetics, PCOS, stress levels, sleep quality, age, oestrogen levels and muscle mass. How you deal with glucose is multifaceted and depends on your current physical state.

Whatever the cause, a glucose spike makes your body signal the pancreas to send insulin, which removes glucose from the bloodstream. When your body's alarm is set off by a spike in glucose, insulin can go into a frenzy, removing too much glucose from the bloodstream and causing a significant drop that results in low blood sugar. This dip can leave you feeling "hangry", fatigued, and mentally foggy.

As we learnt in chapter 2, if we stay on this roller coaster ride our cells become less effective at communicating and, eventually, resistant to insulin. Your ability to manage glucose also drops when oestrogen is low, such as during the hormonal shifts of perimenopause and menopause, as oestrogen can improve glucose sensitivity.

MANAGING GLUCOSE SPIKES

So, what can be done? I find it helps to think of your body as a space where nutrients should enter in the right order and balance. Glucose, your body's primary energy source, should arrive "fashionably late" – that way, it has less opportunity to overwhelm your system and trigger a spike.

If fibre arrives first, followed by protein and fat, the digestive system can handle the incoming glucose more effectively than if you were to eat carbohydrates first, on an empty stomach. That's because fibre creates a protective lining in your digestive tract, slowing down glucose absorption, while fat and protein slow down glucose even further, as your digestive system is no longer focused solwly on breaking down starch. That way, by the time glucose arrives, it won't have the same easy access to your bloodstream. This is the level of blood sugar after eating, known as your postprandial glucose level. With other nutrients physically in the way, glucose enters more gradually, keeping blood sugar levels stable.

In other words, the order in which you eat matters. Starting a meal with vegetables or a side salad creates a barrier in the digestive tract. When dining out, try beginning with vegetables or a side salad before your main meal. Then pair your starch with some protein and fat to ensure glucose arrives "fashionably late".

The same rule applies to breakfast. How you start your day sets the tone for your blood sugar regulation throughout the day, either giving you sustained energy or leading to cravings and energy dips. If you can get breakfast right, you'll set yourself up for success and swerve the blood sugar roller coaster.

Think about what you're eating, and whether it's balanced. Is it a naked carb like a solitary pastry, which could lead to a blood sugar spike? Or is it a starch paired with protein, fat, and fibre for a steadier release of energy, like porridge, or a smoothie (see p.133)?

STYLING YOUR STARCHES

When it comes to nutrition, it's not just about the calories in your meal, but how your food is styled. Even if two meals have the same number of calories, the way they are structured can lead to two very different biochemical responses in your body. One meal might spike your blood glucose, while the other might keep it stable. This is why calorie counting is an outdated approach – it oversimplifies the value of food and ignores how different food structures impact your body on a biochemical level. Every time you eat, ask yourself these two questions:

WHERE IS THE PROTEIN?
WHERE IS THE FAT?

When you've got starch on your plate, every meal should be styled with these two macronutrients. With the added workout that protein and fat provide, fewer glucose bonds are broken and, as a result, less glucose enters your bloodstream, preventing your body from sounding the glucose alarm.

MEAL FORMULAS

Instead of having a plain piece of sourdough for breakfast with a dollop of jam, style your starch (sourdough) with a poached egg, half an avocado, and a handful of spinach. These two meals both feature the same central ingredient, but will trigger very different biochemical responses in the body.

Let's look at another common breakfast: porridge. Oats are great, but pair them with the wrong ingredients, and you could be welcoming a potential spike. Porridge with honey is simply starch paired with sugar.

Instead, "style" your porridge (oatmeal) with additions that provide plenty of added healthy fats and protein: think chia seeds, flaxseeds, and nut butter, good-quality vegan protein powder, collagen powder, or a dollop of high-protein yoghurt. Top with colourful berries for sweetness and fibre, instead of adding sugar. Apply the same framework for a smoothie, ensuring there is both a protein and fat.

Whether you take one week or two to introduce the framework in this first pillar, focus on creating three meals a day using the equation below as a guide. Let's keep it simple.

STARCH + PROTEIN + GOOD FAT
=
YOUR NEW FAVOURITE EQUATION

EATING WELL

Aim for three meals a day while minimising snacking; grazing can lead to frequent spikes in insulin levels, which we want to avoid. For most people, unless you are pregnant or breastfeeding, snacking isn't necessary. By spacing out your meals, you will allow your digestive system to rest, reducing unnecessary energy intake and keeping insulin levels stable. If afternoon hunger strikes, consider what you ate at lunch. Did you eat enough protein? Have you been drinking enough water?

Consuming less glucose and styling your food will help stabilize blood sugar, giving you sustained energy, curbing cravings, reducing brain fog and creating a happier home for your hormones by improving your insulin sensitivity.

Finally, remember that macronutrients don't operate absolutes; their interactions are multifaceted. Some foods contain a mix of macronutrients. While beans and legumes are primarily carbohydrates, they also contain protein. Meanwhile, foods we might consider to be primarily protein, like nuts, seeds and oily fish, are also good sources of fat. Many vegetables provide fibre without being starchy. Food structure isn't always black and white.

o   Include protein and healthy fats in your
    meals to stay on the right track.

o   Maximize complex carbs like beans,
    legumes, and starchy vegetables,
    which will deliver glucose into your
    bloodstream at steadier and slower rates.

o   Minimize simple sugars, sweets,
    chocolates, and added refined sugar.
    Simple sugars are responsible for sudden
    and dramatic glucose spikes in your
    bloodstream, which require insulin and
    can lead to insulin resistance. This drives
    hormone imbalance, inflammation, and
    unhealthy weight gain.

o   Remember to style your starches by
    asking yourself, at every meal: "Where
    is the protein? Where is the fat?" This
    supports the efficient digestion of all
    three macronutrients.

o   Eat three meals a day to minimize the
    urge to snack, which can spike glucose
    levels. Do not skip breakfast.

HOW TO STYLE STARCH

Styling food the right way, incorporating protein and good fats alongside carbohydrates, will keep your blood sugar stable and your hormones balanced.

✹ A source of both carbohydrate and protein

✦ A source of both protein and fat

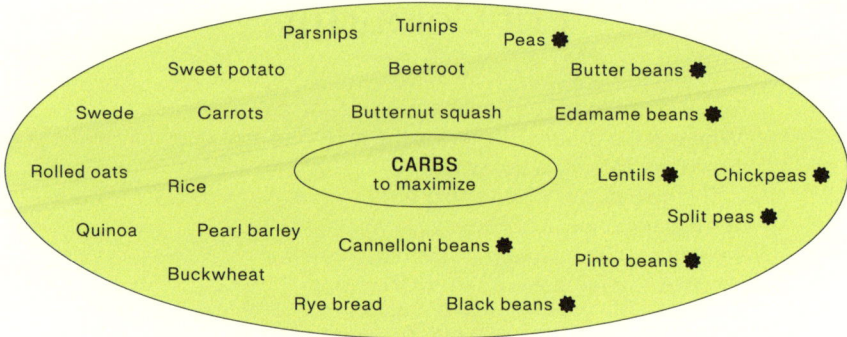

+

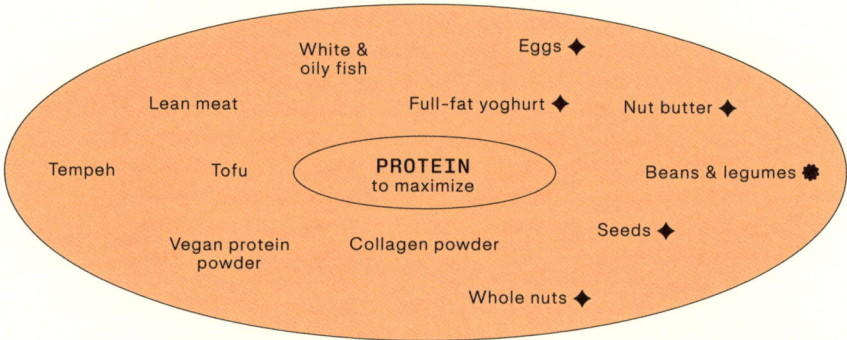

+

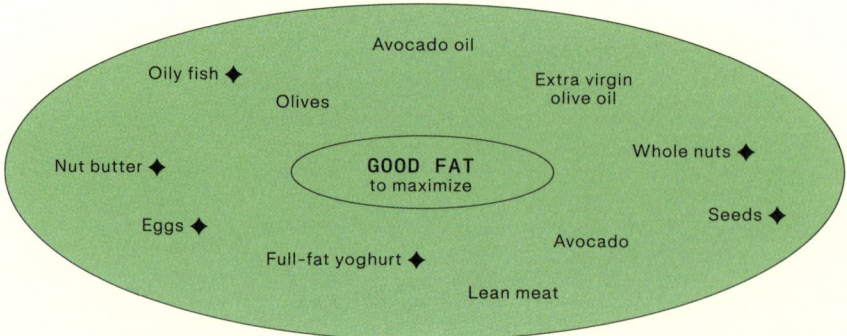

=

A STYLED STARCH

Pillar Two
Eat Colourful

You've learnt to take a beat before you eat, asking yourself, "Where is the protein? Where is the fat?" The next question should be: "Where is the colour?"

The goal of this pillar is to create a more balanced, low-inflammation environment for your hormones. As we've seen, diet-induced inflammation is a prime cause of hormone dysfunction (see p.107).

THE POWER OF DIVERSITY

Nurturing a positive approach to food is about focusing on what to add – not what to restrict. Colourful, bioactive nutritive molecules are a great way to begin. Diversity is key – the more colour, the better! Plant-based foods high in vitamins and minerals are colourful because they contain phytochemicals, which are natural compounds that give plants their colour, taste, and aroma. They also support the hundreds of pathways comprising your hormonal landscape, and your gut and vaginal microbiome, and are vital in boosting the Omega 3-to-6 ratio (see p.138) and liver detoxification.

MINIMIZING INFLAMMATION

Using colour to reduce inflammation is easy – it comes down to increasing:

Phytonutrients – found in plant-based foods like fruits, vegetables, and herbs

Antioxidants – found in foods rich in antioxidant compounds, like berries, nuts, and leafy greens

Raw materials for your hormones to thrive – including healthy fats, amino acids, probiotics, vitamins, and minerals

> **THE OMEGA 3-TO-6 RATIO**
> The Omega 3-to-6 ratio is a fine balance. A diet rich in Omega-3 is better for our hormone health, while an imbalance with excessive Omega-6 can encourage inflammation.

Bolstering your diet in these three ways will nourish and populate your gut microbiome, as well as stabilize your vaginal microbiome. And, of course, there's the bonus of enjoying a beautiful, colourful plate of food.

Maximizing fibre-rich, plant-based whole foods that are colourful and full of vitamins and minerals will support your nutrition and make you feel wonderful.

Don't count calories – count your colours instead.

THE POWER OF NUTRIENTS

Food is more than just an energy source. The nutrients in your food can give your body and hormones the essential materials to function optimally, helping the millions of biological pathways in action every millisecond, nourishing and feeding your gut and vaginal microbiome, and defending you from disease and free-radical damage.

Nutrients are fundamental, especially at significant life stages like puberty, pregnancy, postpartum, perimenopause, and beyond. Even for you to understand this sentence, vitamin B12 must be adequately maintaining your myelin sheaths, which surround the nerve cells in your brain and allow electrical impulses to travel from one nerve cell to the next.

Magnesium is brilliant at regulating mood in puberty. The vitamin E found in avocados is fantastic for your skin health. Berries, rich in antioxidants, are highly beneficial when you are trying to conceive and for foetal development during pregnancy. The phytoestrogens found in tofu and edamame beans can alleviate hot flushes during menopause.

PREGNANCY AND NUTRITIONAL DEPLETION

Pregnancy and the postpartum period can put you into a nutritional overdraft. During the hormonal shift of pregnancy, the impact on your nutrient stores is enormous. Your body will prioritize the new life, ensuring they get everything they need through the placenta (and, later, via breastfeeding if you choose to do so). As a result, you can be left with the nutritional scraps.

This nutrient deficit can express itself as low energy or mood, and feelings of complete exhaustion due to low levels of iron, B vitamins, Omega-3, vitamin D, zinc, and selenium

This is a harsh backdrop for the incoming hormonal shifts of the postnatal period – without intervention, the female body can take years to get back to pre-baby nutrient levels. Throw in another baby or two, and you're looking at a long stint of life in a potential nutrient deficit.

Pregnancy can be especially hard on your iron and Omega-3 stores. As blood volume increases during pregnancy, so too do your iron requirements. It is vital to increase your iron intake at this time. Falling into a state of iron deficiency can be harmful to your long-term fertility and even leave you at risk of postnatal depression – a condition that many studies have linked to diminished levels of nutrients such as Omega-3.

PUTTING COLOUR INTO ACTION

By consistently increasing your fibre, vitamins, minerals, and phytonutrients, you can positively change your hormonal picture – reducing inflammation, keeping insulin balanced, increasing your nutrient status, nourishing your microbiomes, and bringing you joy.

By "colour", I mean the vast, vibrant array of plant-derived foods including vegetables, fruits, herbs and spices, nuts, teas, wholegrains, beans, and legumes. The kaleidoscope of colour in these foods comes down to their structure and phytochemicals. The colour of plants, vegetables, and fruit is determined by their structure, which reflects certain wavelengths of light while absorbing others.

The rich yellow, orange, and red hues found in butternut squash, carrots, peppers, and pumpkins, for example, are thanks to the molecule structure of carotenoids. Carotenoids are packed with antioxidants. Each colour in our food brings its own unique benefits, which is why it's essential to have as many colours on your plate as possible.

I guarantee that, most of the time, you can find more colour to add. You might have a random bell pepper sitting in the fridge, or some cucumber, courgette (zucchini), carrot, or red cabbage you can dice up, grate, and use to garnish. It doesn't have to be complicated or glamorous. Simple beetroots (beets) and carrots count just as much as heritage (heirloom) tomatoes or purple-sprouting broccoli. This is about having fun and inviting added colour into your world.

It's time to meet your micronutrients, minerals, and vitamins, as well as your phytonutrients. These are the chemicals that plants produce to protect themselves. In addition to this, they also protect our own health.

We're told we need all four, but what exactly are they – and why do they matter?

PHYTONUTRIENTS

Phytonutrients, also known as phytochemicals, are vital compounds found in plant-based foods. They can help enrich your starches with colourful, fibre-rich ingredients and essential micronutrients.

WEEKDAY RAINBOW CHECKLIST

Create a rainbow every week with
colourful, plant-based foods that add
variety to your plate.

RED

Examples:	Phytonutrients:	Health benefits:
Cherries, apples, raspberries, strawberries, watermelon, beetroot, radishes, rhubarb	Carotenoids, lycopenes, olyphenols and anthocyanins	Prevent cancer and improve cardiovascular health

DAY   1 ◯   2 ◯   3 ◯   4 ◯   5 ◯

ORANGE

Examples:	Phytonutrients	Health benefits
Apricots, orange bell peppers, butternut squash, cantaloupes, carrots, mangoes, nectarines	Carotenoids, beta and alpha carotene	Healthy heart, vision and immune system

DAY   1 ◯   2 ◯   3 ◯   4 ◯   5 ◯

YELLOW

Examples:	Phytonutrients:	Health benefits:
Yellow bell peppers, sweetcorn, lemons, squash, swedes, star fruit, pineapple, squash	Carotenoids, lycopenes, olyphenols and anthocyanins	Healthy heart, vision, and immune system

DAY   1 ◯   2 ◯   3 ◯   4 ◯   5 ◯

GREEN

Examples:	Phytonutrients:	Health benefits:
Asparagus, avocados, green bell peppers, broccoli, courgette, cabbage, celery	Carotenoids, zeaxanthin, lutein	For good vision and prevention of age-related macular degeneration

DAY   1 ◯   2 ◯   3 ◯   4 ◯   5 ◯

PURPLE / BLUE

Examples:	Phytonutrients:	Health benefits:
Blackberries, blackcurrants, blueberries, red cabbage, purple carrots, aubergines	Anthocyanins	Help improve memory, healthy aging, and urinary tract health

DAY   1 ◯   2 ◯   3 ◯   4 ◯   5 ◯

WHITE

Examples:	Phytonutrients:	Health benefits:
Butter beans, cauliflower, cannellini beans, chickpeas, garlic, white onion, shallots	Allylic sulphides or alliums	Prevent against carcinogens causing stomach cancer, and lower cholesterol

DAY   1 ◯   2 ◯   3 ◯   4 ◯   5 ◯

While macronutrients (see p.125) provide energy, phytonutrients are non-nutritive compounds, delivering valuable protective health properties – particularly for your hormone health and oestrogen clearance. There is substantial evidence showing how effective phytonutrients are in preventing menopausal symptoms, as well as cancer, cardiovascular disease, diabetes, osteoporosis, gastrointestinal disorders, atopic eczema, and hyperactivity, and well as gynaecological, neurological, and immunological disorders.

Many colourful phytonutrients are also antioxidants (see p.144). They are anti-inflammatory and play a pivotal role in your immune system, hormone metabolism, and heart and brain health. Phytonutrients support your detoxification by reducing DNA damage, regulating the cell cycle, and interacting with and even mimicking your hormones.

Now we'll explore a few of the most important phytonutrients, and the colourful foods that contain them.

PHYTOESTROGENS

It is crucial to incorporate phytoestrogens, plant compounds structurally similar to oestriadol, during menopause.

OESTROGEN AND PHYTOESTROGEN

Classified as flavonoids, lignans, or stilbenes, phytoestrogens can have pro- or anti-oestrogenic effects by binding to oestrogen receptors. When oestrogen levels drop, unoccupied receptors disrupt the body's processes. Phytoestrogens, though weaker than actual oestrogen, bind to these receptors, helping restore balance and easing low oestrogen effects.

TOP SOURCES OF PHYTOESTROGENS:

Edamame	Beans and legumes
Tofu	Ground flaxseeds
Tempeh	Sesame seeds
Organic, non-GMO soy	Garlic
Broccoli	

CAROTENOIDS

Carotenoid phytonutrients are present in red, orange, yellow, and a few green vegetables. The most important carotenoid subcategories I recommend you maximize are beta-carotene and lycopene. Foods containing these are rich in vitamin A and vitamin C (see pp.148–49), and contain properties that can potentially decrease the risk of certain cancers.

TOP SOURCES OF CAROTENOIDS:

Butternut squash	Sweet potato
Pumpkin	Carrots
Tomato	Spinach
Grapefruit	Kale

Cooking your vegetables can "free up" carotenoids, making them more available to convert to pre-formed vitamin A (see p.146). Cooking butternut squash and carrots will help your body digest and receive their full nutritional benefit, as will styling them with a good source of fat like seeds or extra virgin olive oil.

To increase your intake of carotenoids, look no further than the trusty tomato. With an antioxidant activity exceeding alpha and beta carotene, tomatoes play a big part in our nutritional intake. Famed for their protective role in the prostate (get any men in your life onto tomatoes pronto!), new research also speaks highly of tomatoes' role in women's metabolic health – particularly for postmenopausal women.

Rich in beta-carotenoids and lycopene, a recent, randomized study investigating the impact of a diet rich in tomatoes on metabolic health in postmenopausal women found that it led to significantly lower cholesterol, lower blood pressure, and lower blood sugar. The study concluded that consuming fresh tomatoes can increase antioxidant biomarkers, reducing the risk of metabolic syndrome in postmenopausal women.

ANTIOXIDANTS

Antioxidants neutralize free radicals – they are literally "anti" oxidative stress (see p.76). Free radicals are created in the body by certain foods, types of exercise, or exposure to toxins. They're bad news for many reasons, especially when they gang up together and outnumber your antioxidants, which can lead to oxidative stress. As we learnt in chapter 2, oxidative stress occurs when there's an imbalance between free radicals and antioxidants in the body, causing damage to cells, tissues, and DNA. Antioxidants work by stabilizing free radicals, either donating an electron or taking one away from the free radical, leaving it with an even number of electrons. This helps create a stable environment for your hormones to thrive, protecting areas like the gut from free radical damage. Think of antioxidants like roving scavengers out to protect you – your only job is to keep upping your antioxidant levels by eating more colourful foods.

TOP SOURCES OF ANTIOXIDANTS:

Blueberries, strawberries, and raspberries	Artichokes
Pecans	Kale and spinach

VITAMINS

Vitamins and minerals are the co-factors and coenzymes for your hormones and metabolism, essential to nearly every bodily pathway and process. For this system to work, along with all your body's biological and protective actions, vitamins and minerals must be present. The actions may be left incomplete or void if vitamins and minerals are absent. Vitamins are found in many different foods, but must be converted into another form with the presence of minerals like zinc (see p.153).

With a food industry geared towards ultra-processed mass production, most people are not getting enough vitamins and minerals. Soil quality is also declining worldwide, and since soil provides essential nutrients for plants, poorer soil leads to crops with a lower nutrient value.

PERIMENOPAUSE, MENOPAUSE, AND PHYTOESTROGENS

By increasing your intake of phytoestrogens, you can improve symptoms of perimenopause and menopause such as hot flushes. Fascinatingly, research has also shown that in Japan, where consumption of good quality soya (soy) products is high, there are fewer menopausal symptoms reported – particularly hot flushes – compared to women in Western countries, and lower rates of breast cancer, which we are at greater risk of as we age. Observational studies in Japan show an approximate 30 per cent reduction in risk. The effect was greatest for those who ate a large amount of soy products during childhood and adolescence, which means that it could be especially beneficial for teens to include plenty of tofu in their diet to safeguard their long-term health.

When looking at combining phytoestrogens with hormonotherapy (hormone therapy), such as through Tamoxifen, results have been controversial. Some reports even suggest that phytoestrogens may interfere with the effects of anti-cancer drugs.

145

Bodily shifts during puberty, pregnancy, postnatal, perimenopause, and beyond involving rapid growth, high stress, or changes to your menstruation cycle or hormones will make you especially vulnerable during a vitamin or mineral deficiency. These are times at which it is even more important to seek out a vitamin-rich diet.

Vitamins are either fat- or water-soluble. Fat-soluble vitamins (A, D, E, K) require dietary fat for absorption, so a low-fat diet may impact their uptake. Unlike fat-soluble vitamins, which are stored in the body for later use, vitamin C and those in the B family (such as B2 and B12) are water-soluble, meaning your body eliminates any excess through urine. Ever had your pee turn a luminous yellow after taking vitamin supplements? That's a sign that you're taking too many costly water-soluble supplements – it's literally money down the drain!

PROVITAMIN VITAMIN A VERSUS PRE-FORMED VITAMIN A

Vitamin A comes in two forms: pre-formed vitamin A, found as retinol in organ meat such as liver, fish oil, and other fortified foods, and provitamin A, which is the form found in carotenoids.

Pre-formed vitamin A arrives readily usable for your body, but can be toxic in excess as it bypasses your body's conversion process. A fat-soluble vitamin, pre-formed vitamin A cannot be excreted via urine, but must be absorbed with an added fat (see p.95). Pregnant women or those trying to conceive should be cautious of this vitamin, which can harm foetal development – avoid high-dose supplements or excessive amounts of organ meat.

Provitamin A, on the other hand, needs to be converted by the body to an active form by metabolizing with retinol, retinaldehyde, and retinoic acid. This form of vitamin A is a crucial micronutrient for pregnant women and foetuses. There's no danger of over-eating provitamin A if you're getting it through vegetables, so embrace carrots, squash, and sweet potato.

VITAMIN D

Vitamin D supports your reproductive and bone health, skeletal muscle, immune system, and glucose balance. Sunshine helps our bodies to synthesize vitamin D, but given that many people don't have access to year-round sunshine, it's worth investing in a good vitamin D supplement.

Vitamin D can control gene expression and act as a hormone. It should be at the top of your radar for hormone health because vitamin D deficiency can drive dysfunction – and low vitamin D levels are widespread. Vitamin D deficiency is prevalent in women with PCOS, with about 67–85 per cent of women experiencing low levels. Vitamin D deficiency may even exacerbate the symptoms of PCOS, with observational studies showing lower levels of circulating vitamin D were associated with insulin resistance, ovulatory and menstrual irregularities, lower rates of pregnancy, hirsutism, hyperandrogenism, obesity, and elevated cardiovascular disease risk factors.

Menopausal women are at risk of reduced bone density and increased risk of fracture due to a decline in oestrogen levels, making osteoporosis a significant risk factor. Vitamin D is key to maintaining calcium homeostasis and bone metabolism, making this is a vitamin you should be mindful of and, in most cases, supplement.

It can be hard to source the necessary amount of vitamin D from food sources alone; it is contained in oily fish, eggs, butter, and mushrooms, but only in modest amounts. Therefore, this is one vitamin I recommend you take an additional supplement of about 2,000iu daily.

THE VITAMIN B FAMILY

The B vitamins boost and serve as vital cofactors throughout the body. Deficiency can have serious physical and psychological effects. Closely tied to your sex hormones, B vitamins influence reproductive health. Women who are pregnant or trying to conceive require even higher levels of B vitamins such as folate.

B vitamins include B1 (thiamine), B2 (riboflavin), B3 (niacin), and B5 (pantothenic acid). Of particular importance to your hormones, B6 (pyridoxine), B9 (folate), and B12 (cobalamin) work together as a trio. They support hormone regulation, cell metabolism, energy production, your brain, and your central nervous system.

B6 PYRIDOXINE

B6 plays a key role in balancing your blood sugar balance. It it is the cofactor of an enzyme that releases glucose from glycogen. It helps regulate your sex hormones. Signs of deficiency include acne, PMS symptoms, fluid retention, nausea, and breast soreness.

VITAMIN A

Vitamin A helps to regulate and control gene expression. This vitamin supports your eye health, reproduction, and cell renewal. It works wonders for your skin health and immune system, and influences your thyroid hormone metabolism and progesterone production.

Vitamin A deficiency is closely linked to thyroid gland damage and reduced function. Research suggests that it has a meaningful impact on thyroid structure, function, and hormonal balance. Vitamin A deficiency is also often associated with iodine deficiency, a significant driver of hypothyroidism (see p.71).

TOP SOURCES OF VITAMIN A:*

Pre-formed vitamin A: liver, egg yolks, fish, liver, butter, whole milk

Carrots

Kale

Butternut squash

Mango

Spinach

Pumpkin

VITAMIN E

Vitamin E is a wonderful antioxidant that safeguards your skin, eyes, and immunity. It has also been shown to have positive effects on PMS, reducing symptoms of anxiety, pain, cravings, and low mood.

TOP SOURCES OF VITAMIN E:*

Sunflower seeds

Pumpkin seeds

Green leafy vegetables

Avocados

Pine nuts

Almonds

Hazelnuts

*sources include, but are not limited to, this list

VITAMIN C

Vitamin C is a key antioxidant and immunity superhero. It supports progesterone production, which is essential for your adrenal glands. These adrenal glands produce hormones that help regulate your stress response, metabolism, and blood pressure, among other vital bodily functions.

Crucial to the biosynthesis of collagen, L–carnitine, and certain neurotransmitters, vitamin C is also involved in protein metabolism.

TOP SOURCES OF VITAMIN C:*

Kiwis

Red peppers

Blackcurrants and redcurrants

Citrus fruits

Papaya

Strawberries

Raspberries

Kale

Watercress

Pineapple

VITAMIN K

Vitamin K safeguards blood clotting and bones, and functions as a coenzyme (see p.144) when your body synthesizes proteins involved in blood coagulation and bone metabolism. Vitamin K can help improve bone health and reduce the risk of bone fractures, especially in postmenopausal women, making this an especially useful vitamin to supplement in later life stages.

TOP SOURCES OF VITAMIN K:*

Spinach

Spring greens

Sprouts

B9 FOLATE

You may have heard how important folic acid is in the lead-up to pregnancy. It is recommended that women hoping to become pregnant supplement with 400mcg of folic acid, a synthetic form of B9 folate. Folate is the natural form of B9 found in foods such as dark green leafy vegetables. It must then be converted into its active form, methylfolate (5-MTHF). Choose supplements carefully – opting for folate or methylfolate might be beneficial, as some people cannot convert folate due to the MTHF gene.

B12 COBALAMIN

Think neurological support and conception! Cobalamin's most bioavailable form comes from animal products, so if you are vegan or eat mainly plant-based food, you must monitor your levels and supplement. B12 deficiency can significantly impact fertility.

TOP SOURCES OF VITAMIN B:*

Green leafy vegetables	Mushrooms
Nuts	Meat
Seeds	Fish
Beans	Eggs
Legumes	Dairy products

MINERALS

Minerals are the essential nutrients that your body needs to properly function. Minerals such as calcium, magnesium and iron help with processes such as building bones, transmitting nerve signals, and producing energy.

Minerals work in tandem with vitamins, either aiding bioavailability or hindering it. Vitamin D, for example, helps the body absorb calcium from food, especially plant sources like leafy greens. Vitamin C helps the body absorb iron, especially non-heme (plant-based) iron from foods such as beans and lentils. Zinc can block the body's ability to absorb copper.

MAGNESIUM

Responsible for hormone balance, sleep, and muscle support, magnesium is your central nervous system's best friend and can help combat anxiety. Magnesium citrate is a supplement that helps with bowel movements and constipation, and magnesium glycinate supports your sleep. If you're deficient in magnesium, you might experience twitching around your eyes, anxiety, or constipation.

TOP SOURCES OF MAGNESIUM:*

Dark green leafy vegetables

Pumpkin seeds

Chia seeds

Edamame beans

Almonds

CALCIUM

This vital mineral supports your bones, muscles, and blood clotting, safeguarding your cardiac function and acting as an enzymatic signal in biochemical pathways. Your bones are well-stocked with calcium, but if levels get low, your body will steal it from your bones to maintain steady levels in the blood and support other critical functions in the body. This is especially risky during menopause, when your bone density is compromised by declining oestrogen.

TOP SOURCES OF CALCIUM:*

Sardines (bones and all!)

Full-fat yoghurt

Cottage cheese

Firm tofu

Leafy green veg

Beans

Legumes

Salmon

*sources include, but are not limited to, this list

IODINE

Closely connected to your thyroid, your thyroid hormones are composed of ions of iodine. It is an essential component of your thyroid hormones, thyroxine (T4) and triiodothyronine (T3). A large number of hypothyroid cases are linked to iodine deficiency.

TOP SOURCES OF IODINE:*

Seaweed

Cottage cheese

Cod

Full-fat yoghurt

IRON

Iron supports your DNA synthesis, thyroid hormones, circulation, brain health, and the transportation of oxygen around the body. Signs of deficiency include fatigue, dizziness, shortness of breath, hair loss, cold hands and feet, pale skin, or concave nails.

Vegetarian sources of iron (non heme) aren't that well absorbed by the body compared to animal sources of iron (heme), but adding vitamin C helps absorption, so style any iron-rich veggies with a squeeze of lemon, plus a side of bell peppers or sweet potato.

Iron levels can drop during puberty due to rapid growth and via menstrual blood loss. Pregnant women are also at risk of iron deficiency due to the increased requirement for iron within the body. If there is an increase in heavy bleeding during perimenopause, women may be at risk of deficiency due to menstrual blood loss.

TOP SOURCES OF IRON:*

Red meat

Green leafy veg

Nuts and seeds

Legumes

Dried apricots

Eggs

*sources include, but are not limited to, this list

Zinc safeguards your skin, immunity, reproductive system, and sense of taste and smell, maintaining the structure of cell membranes and protecting them from oxidative damage.

Signs of deficiency include skin conditions such as eczema, acne, poor wound healing, hair loss, and low libido. Zinc and copper compete for absorption in the body, so if you have a copper IUD, you may want to maximize zinc-rich foods. If you are taking or coming off the oral contraceptive pill, remember that oral contraceptives often increase levels of copper and decrease zinc.

TOP SOURCES OF ZINC:*

Oysters

Shellfish

Pumpkin seeds

Nuts

Legumes

Selenium is responsible for your thyroid hormones, converting inactive thyroxine (T4) into active triiodothyronine (T3), supporting thyroid function, reproduction, and immunity – you also require more when pregnant or breastfeeding. Signs of deficiency include a weakened immune system, brittle nails, hair loss, and cognitive decline. Oral contraceptives can lower your selenium levels, so you may want to take a supplement if you're taking the pill.

TOP SOURCES OF SELENIUM:*

Full-fat yoghurt

Pork

Beef

Turkey

Chicken

Fish

Shellfish

Eggs

Brazil nuts (Eat no more than three a day as they contain almost twice your daily selenium intake.)

Like vitamins, minerals act as essential cofactors in numerous pathways and functions within the body, assisting in the smooth transfer of signals and processes. Let's look at a few of them more closely.

ELECTROLYTES

Electrolytes include minerals such as sodium, potassium, chloride, magnesium, calcium, phosphate, and bicarbonates. These ions maintain the volume of bodily fluids, blood, pressure and nerve conduction. They are important cofactors for many pathways and enzymatic reactions, which can impact your overall hormone balance and fertility. Where there is an electrolyte imbalance, follicular fluid compositions can be altered leading to a restriction of follicular growth.

Electrolyte ions maintain the volume of bodily fluids and blood pressure, playing a key role in muscle contractions and nerve signalling and are essential for enzymatic reactions such as digestion and energy production.

Sodium, for instance, is linked to oestrogen synthesis because it supports the processes that regulate hormone production. Sodium, potassium, and calcium are also all linked to the contraction and relaxation of the uterus during a period – calcium triggers the muscle contractions that help shed the uterine lining while sodium and potassium work together to keep the muscles functioning properly. Calcium can also activate an immature egg (oocyte) to become a mature egg (ovum). An imbalance of oocyte electrolytes can adversely affect fertility.

Although electrolytes are found in food, it can still be beneficial to boost your levels. Try mixing 2.5ml (0.088 fl oz) of electrolytes, in liquid or sachet form, with your morning water after breakfast. It goes without saying, of course, that we should drink about two litres (4.23 pints) of filtered water daily, occasionally adding electrolytes to support hormone health.

ADAPTOGENIC HERBS AND SPICES

Boosting colour for your nutritional intake goes beyond fruit and veg. Herbs and spices are wonderful additions, too. Adaptogens are a class of herbs, roots, and mushrooms that can lower cortisol levels by increasing the enzyme that converts cortisol to cortisone, which is an inactive hormone with anti-inflammatory properties. Adaptogens also exert a stress-soothing effect by promoting balance in the body through several mechanisms that regulate the hypothalamic-pituitary-adrenal (HPA) axis.

MACA ROOT

Maca is a fabulous source of B2, iron, calcium, and flavonoids, and can promote antioxidants in the body. Studies have shown it to be a valuable non-hormonal plant for balancing hormones and alleviating menopausal symptoms such as hot flushes, sexual dysfunction, night sweating, interrupted sleep, nervousness, depression, and heart palpitations. Mood- and libido-boosting, try adding 3–5g (0.10–0.18 oz) to a morning smoothie. Maca is not advised for those with thyroid dysfunction and is best avoided when undergoing treatments that modify hormonal levels, such as those prescribed for breast cancer.

SAGE

Sage is an incredible antimicrobial, antioxidant, and anti-inflammatory herb. Delicious cooked, it's also wonderful as a tea. It can help suppress hot flushes in perimenopause and menopause. Take particular caution if you are pregnant or breastfeeding.

ASHWAGANDHA ROOT

Ashwagandha is anti-inflammatory as well as adaptogenic. Studies show that supplementing this root extract significantly reduces stress and can improve overall quality of life. Add 3–5g (0.10–0.18 oz) of the dried root to a smoothie. Take particular care if you are pregnant or breastfeeding, as ashwagandha may cause uterine contractions. Its full effects on breastfeeding women are not yet fully understood.

TURMERIC

Turmeric can be wonderful for endometriosis. Famed for its anti-inflammatory properties, it supports your hormones and brain health thanks to a compound called curcumin, a powerhouse that can also support liver detoxification. Boost your intake by adding it to curries, soups, scrambled eggs, scrambled tofu, lattes, and sauces. Combine it with black pepper (to aid absorption) and a little extra virgin olive oil or MCT oil to maximize turmeric's benefits. You'd need to consume a lot of turmeric to get the full benefits, so taking a turmeric supplement of around 500mg (0.018 oz) daily while integrating it into your diet is the best approach.

AGNUS CASTUS

Also known as chasteberry, agnus castus has demonstrated efficacy in relieving PMS and breast pain. It can be used as a low-dose tincture if coming off the oral contraceptive pill to support the luteal phase and boost progesterone levels, to enhance the corpus luteum. Agnus castus has been shown to increase progesterone, which can be beneficial during perimenopause and menopause. Be aware that it should be avoided if taking HRT. Take special caution if pregnant or breastfeeding.

GINGER

An anti-inflammatory root, ginger is also wonderful for nausea – particularly during pregnancy. Grate it into dishes like salads, or slice ginger into hot water to make fresh ginger tea.

CINNAMON

Cinnamon enhances insulin efficiency and supports blood sugar regulation. It is a great spice to add to breakfast bowls, overnight chia seed pudding, and hot drinks. It's also an antifungal herb, which is anti-candida, a yeast that can overgrow and cause thrush (yeast infections), fatigue, and digestive issues.

COLOUR

sliced or grated – carrot, courgette (zucchini), cucumber, red cabbage, red onion, celery, peppers, cauliflower, broccoli, broccoli sprouts, garlic, fermented foods (like sauerkraut, kimchi, live fermented pickled vegetables), grated apples, pomegranates, radishes, tomato, sweetcorn, lemon, asparagus, avocado, green peppers, cabbage, celery, chard, cucumber, green beans, purple carrots, aubergine

+

STARCH = LEGUMES & BEANS / WHOLEGRAIN / STARCHY VEG

lentils, chickpeas, cannellini beans, blacks beans, quinoa, hummus, wild rice, wholegrain rice, edamame beans, buckwheat, pearl barely, sweet potato, butternut squash, roasted beetroot (beet)

+

PROTEIN

salmon fillet, sardines, tuna, eggs, chicken, tofu, tempha, mackerel, grilled turkey, grass-fed steak strips, white fish

+

GREEN LEAVES

spinach, rocket, watercress, lettuce, lamb's lettuce, kale

+

FRESH HERBS

mint, parsley, coriander, basil

+

HEALTHY FAT

avocado, pumpkin seeds, sunflower seeds, tahini, sesame seeds, anchovy, nuts, hemp oil, hemp hearts

+

DRESSING

Try: extra virgin olive oil + fresh lemon juice + white wine vinegar
Vinaigrette: 1 tbsp olive oil, 1 tbsp apple cider vinegar, ½ teaspoon mustard
Tahini: 1 tbsp of tahini, juice of half a lemon, mixed into a paste and adding water for your desired consistency

PILLAR TWO
EAT COLOURFUL
RECAP

o At every meal, ask yourself, "Where is the colour?" There is often room for more. Power clash the colours on your plate – make it joyful!

o Pair any food sources of vitamin D, A, E, and K with a healthy fat to aid absorption.

o Tread with caution, as plants are powerful! They can change your hormonal function and interact with medication. Take extra care when pregnant or breastfeeding. Check the label or consult a qualified healthcare professional.

o Think beyond hydration – add high-quality electrolytes to your water once a week.

o Create a vibrant plate for the various nutrients your hormones need, giving your hormones the raw materials to thrive.

Pillar Three
Eat Smart

The Positive Method is not about restricting your eating, but eating smarter. In the last pillar, we focused on using colour to maximize your intake of vitamins and nutrients. Now, we'll look at the other aspects of your diet that can be tweaked to support systems like your gut microbiome and liver, which can impact your hormone health.

We'll also dive into some hot topics to help you make informed food choices, from navigating ultra-processed foods, calorie counting, dairy, skin health, organic options, reducing alcohol, and choosing the right oils, all to create an environment where your hormones can thrive – by eating smart.

GET TO KNOW YOUR GUT

We've learnt about the gut and vaginal microbiome (see p.87 and p.92) and their role in your hormone health – but how do we nourish them?

Feeding your gut microbiome will create a more diverse colony of gut bacteria and in turn help maintain a healthy vaginal microbiome, which will benefit your reproductive and overall health.

Your gut and vaginal microbiome contain complex biological ecosystems that are in continuous communication with each other. Hormone dysfunction can be exasperated and attributed to an interplay of genetic and environmental factors. There are many ways of influencing and modifying the gut environment, such as having a fibre-rich diet high in prebiotics and probiotics, or taking supplements.

This is your opportunity to influence and improve the condition of your microbiome and your gut lining.

As we discussed on p.87, your gut microbiome is a community that thrives on diversity. To support this diversity, you need to feed your gut microbiome an array of different foods. This involves two types of food in particular: prebiotic and probiotic. Prebiotic foods act as nourishment for the existing bacteria, while probiotic foods introduce new, beneficial bacteria. You can increase both of these through your diet and supplementation.

PREBIOTIC FOODS

Prebiotics are fibre-rich, non-digested food components that feed your gut microbiome. Studies have shown that prebiotics exert a remarkable influence on human health. They can modulate the composition and function of microorganisms that populate your gut – nourishing and feeding your intestinal microbiome. Once the probiotic dietary fibres are broken down and fermented, the end product comprises short-chain fatty acids like butyrate, acetate, and propionate. These molecules are small enough to slip through your gut lining and travel around your bloodstream to organs all over your body. Fabulous prebiotic foods, therefore, positively impact your bacteria and your metabolic and hormone health.

Resistant starch (see p.128) also acts like a prebiotic. As its name suggests, it resists being broken down by human digestive enzymes in the small intestine, and thus ends up fermented in the large intestine, where it feeds all of your lovely gut microbes.

PREBIOTIC FOODS TO MAXIMIZE:

Artichokes	Apples
Asparagus	Avocados
Chicory root	Green bananas
Leafy green vegetables	Berries
Cooked and cooled potatoes	Seaweed
Onions	Beans
Leeks	Legumes
Garlic	Flaxseeds
Tomatoes	Oats

PROBIOTIC FOODS

Probiotics can deliver fresh energy to your gut microbiome by delivering live bacteria. While prebiotics are a food source for the beneficial bacteria in your gut, probiotic foods contain already live bacteria and are a direct source of new life for your microbiome. The living microbes present in probiotic foods can travel to your gut, find a home there, and start multiplying.

Fermented foods are an excellent source of probiotics, as they contain live microorganisms that are created through fermentation – a controlled process of microbial growth and enzymatic action. Adding bacteria to milk, for example, is a way of using fermentation to make live yoghurt. These microorganisms can bring diversity and dynamism to your gut microbiome.

Ideally, try eating three to four kinds of fermented foods a week – think kimchi, sauerkraut, kefir, sourdough bread, and unpasteurized cheese. There are plenty of ways to incorporate these foods into your diet. Kimchi, for instance, goes well with eggs.

By encouraging the amount of *lactobacillus* in your gut, you will also influence and nourish your vaginal microbiome.

PROBIOTIC FOODS TO MAXIMIZE INCLUDE:

Live yoghurt	Miso
Kefir	Sauerkraut
Kimchi	Sourdough bread
Tempeh	Pickles in brine

SYNBIOTICS

With a combination of both probiotic and prebiotic properties, synbiotics help probiotics survive in the gut. A healthy *lactobacillus*-rich vaginal microbiome may even help prevent preterm birth. You can get the benefits of both prebiotics and probiotics, which work hand in hand, by combining them in your diet through synbiotic supplementation.

THE BENEFITS OF BONE BROTH

Alongside your prebiotic and probiotic foods, try increasing your intake of bone broth to boost your gut health. It is easily made at home with leftovers after roasting a chicken – just ensure the chicken is of good quality. In cooler months, a cup of bone broth is a lovely afternoon pick-me-up. When making soup, I always use bone broth as a stock. Slow cooking bones draws out minerals and anti-inflammatory amino acids such as collagen, glycine, and glutamine. These proteins can nourish your intestinal lining and reduce the risk of a leaky gut. Glycine is also brilliant for your happy hormone serotonin, stimulating its production in your gut. In addition, glycine helps create your master tripeptide antioxidant glutathione and secretes GLP-1, a hormone that helps regulate appetite.

SMART CHOICES FOR YOUR LIVER

Your liver plays several key roles in maintaining your hormone health (see p.94), but its most important job is clearing oestrogen once it is no longer needed.

It does so by breaking oestrogen down through biotransformation, converting oestrogen into metabolites that can be excreted through your urine and stool.

If this detoxification process is not working optimally (see p.95), oestrogen can be reabsorbed and reactivated in the body, leading to oestrogen dominance. This can even occur with low oestrogen levels, such as during perimenopause, menopause, or conditions such as PCOS.

There are two phases to ensuring your liver is supported at every stage of biotransformation.

PHASE 1: ENZYMES IN THE LIVER MODIFY OESTROGEN

Avoid speeding up this phase by eating turmeric, garlic, and foods high in magnesium, zinc, and vitamin C. Minimize alcohol, nicotine, and caffeine.

PHASE 2: LIVER MAKES OESTROGEN WATER-SOLUBLE

Support this phase with cruciferous vegetables, turmeric, green tea, and rosemary.

No part of the body exists in isolation. Poor gut health can have a knock-on effect on the liver, as imbalances or issues with your microbiome can drive chronic inflammation, impacting your liver's ability to metabolize and detoxify oestrogen – and other hormones – effectively.

SUPPORTING YOUR LIVER:

Hydrate with two litres (4.23 pints) of filtered water daily	Drink liver-supporting herbal teas like milk thistle
Maximize cruciferous vegetables	Eat choline-rich foods such as eggs
Add 1 tbsp of ground flaxseeds to meals	Limit exposure to plastics
Increase fibre	Support your gut with fermented foods and bone broth
Reduce alcohol	

CHANGING YOUR RELATIONSHIP WITH ALCOHOL

If your liver is busy trying to detoxify alcohol, its attention is not going to be on your hormones. Reducing your alcohol intake can only be beneficial. If you're sober-curious and your hormones are in dire straits, this could be a great time to try it. If you do drink regularly, why not try taking alcohol-free days from Sunday to Thursday? Measuring out alcohol at home is also a smart way of tracking your units.

At parties, I like to order what I call "ghost cocktails" – that is, mocktails that people don't know are mocktails – to stay hydrated and enjoy low-alcohol or alcohol-free evenings. A simple club soda with all the trimmings – freshly sliced lime, lemon, or orange – is refreshing and feels special in and of itself. Alcohol-free options are becoming increasingly ubiquitous – you may be surprised at the many choices that are now available.

CRUCIFEROUS VEGETABLES

One vegetable group that is particularly beneficial to boosting liver health is cruciferous vegetables.

These vegetables are used in the body as biologically active compounds like DIM and indole-3-carbinol, which can support your metabolism and clear oestrogen. Cruciferous vegetables also break down into sulforaphane (SFN), which supports liver function. Sulforphane has been shown to affect the metabolism of glucose and lipids in the liver, improving insulin resistance and helping to clear oestrogen.

For this oestrogen-clearing compound sulforaphane to be created, chop your cruciferous vegetables before cooking. Chopping releases a compound called glucoraphanin, which directly supports liver detoxification. However, this enzyme can be destroyed by heat. Ideally, chop up cruciferous vegetables and put them to one side for 40 minutes – sulforaphane will then have time to form. Once that conversion has happened, you won't lose any nutritional value through cooking.

If you're short on time, sprinkle mustard powder on cooked broccoli to reactivate the conversion of glucoraphanin to sulforaphane. Mustard seeds actually contain a more resilient isoform of myrosinase (an enzyme that helps make sulforaphane) – studies found that adding powdered mustard seeds significantly boosted the formation of sulforaphane in heat-processed broccoli. Half a teaspoon to two teaspoons of mustard powder should do it – I like to call this gunpowder broccoli.

Cruciferous vegetables can boost the availability of certain enzymes in your body, especially CYP1A1 and CYP1A2, which we covered on p.96. Studies show how

164

they can increase these enzymes' activity by 20–40 per cent, helping your body clear oestrogen more effectively.

SMART CRUCIFEROUS VEGETABLES FOR YOUR LIVER:

Broccoli	Pak choy (bok choy)
Cauliflower	Brussels sprouts
Kale	Horseradish
Radish	Watercress
Turnip	Chinese cabbage
Cabbage	Wasabi

PRIORITIZING OMEGA-3 OVER OMEGA-6

Omega-3 and Omega-6 are essential fats that your body cannot make, and must obtain from food.

Omega-3 supports your heart, brain, and metabolism, while Omega-6 provides energy. The difference between them lies in their chemical structure, with the last double bond appearing at different points: Omega-3 has its last double bond three carbons from the end, while Omega-6 has it six carbons away. The ratio of these two fats is important for your hormone health; too much Omega-6 can drive inflammation.

To reduce inflammation and support hormone health, keep on top of your Omega-3. A healthy ratio is around 4:1 (or lower) of Omega-6 to Omega-3. Typical Western diets are often closer to 20:1, which is extremely pro-inflammatory. This is down to the tidal wave of Omega-6 seed oils that have entered the food industry, paired with an underconsumption of Omega-3-rich foods. For instance, the intake of linoleic acid (Omega-6) in the US has nearly doubled over the last century.

MAXIMIZE OMEGA-3-RICH FOODS LIKE:

Oily fish	Walnuts
Grass-fed meats	Flaxseeds
Algae	Chia seeds

Animal sources of Omega-3, like oily fish, give you the active forms (EPA and DHA) that your body needs without converting them from plant-based sources. That's why fish such as salmon, mackerel, anchovies, sardines, and herring are so beneficial. These Omega-3s help balance the fats in your diet, and prevent and reduce inflammation.

GO ORGANIC, WHEN YOU CAN

Whenever possible, I would advise choosing organic foods, especially fruits and vegetables. Non-organic foods are likely treated with endocrine-disrupting chemicals and pesticides, which – as you might expect – can be a hormonal nightmare.

Each year, the Environmental Working Group (EWG) tests a wide range of readily available food items for the presence of pesticides. The EWG is a non-profit organization that researches and advocates for human health and the environment. Every year it analyzes 46 items. In 2024, it highlighted 12 foods that contained worryingly high levels of pesticides:

FRUITS AND VEGETABLES LOADED WITH PESTICIDES:

Strawberries	Nectarines
Spinach	Apples
Kale, collard and mustard greens	Bell and hot peppers
Grapes	Cherries
Peaches	Blueberries
Pears	Green beans

In an ideal world, all food would be organic. Since that isn't the case, it's up to us to buy and eat organic as much as is feasible. That being said, not all fruits and vegetables are widely sold in organic form, while cost can also be a barrier. Make smart choices and informed decisions where you can, but if you have to buy non-organic, all is not lost.

Whenever you bring home fruit and vegetables, wash them in a sink filled with one teaspoon of bicarbonate of soda to every two cups of cold water. Soak for about 10 minutes, then rinse everything thoroughly with running water. This should help remove any traces of pesticide. Peeling can also help.

SMART EATING FOR HORMONAL SKIN

As any teenager knows only too well, hormones play a major role in the health and appearance of our skin, and any imbalances can have a very visible effect. Oestrogen, for instance, can impact your skin texture, and the drop in oestrogen levels during the menopause has a profound impact on skin's elasticity, thickness, and collagen content. Cortisol, meanwhile, can drive the expression of inflammatory skin conditions like eczema. Testosterone can drive acne. The appearance of your skin can even change throughout your menstrual cycle.

To support your skin, maximize healthy fats like olive oil, oily fish, nuts, and seeds, vitamin E-rich foods such as avocados, and vitamin A-rich foods like carrots and squash. And of course, the best first step is to keep your skin well hydrated by drinking plenty of water – between six to eight cups a day.

SUPPORTING HORMONAL ACNE

Acne, a chronic inflammatory skin disease of sebaceous follicles, is one of the most common skin disorders. It is typically driven by inflammation and high androgen levels, which are hormones like testosterone, DHEA-S, and DHT that are linked to male sexual characteristics. Testosterone and DHEA-S levels often serve as markers of acne severity. Sleep deprivation and stress can significantly worsen acne by increasing the production of cortisol, which can drive inflammation and increased sebum production in the skin, making it oilier and more prone to breakouts.

Acne is usually more prevalent in teenagers, but in reality, it can strike at any age. If you're suffering from acne alongside excessive hair loss or hair growth, it might be a case of bringing down your levels of DHT. While testosterone and DHT play clear roles in the development of acne, research on the role of oestrogen is ongoing.

There is rarely one single cause driving acne. Alongside hormones, genetics also play a big role in your propensity to acne. While you can try to get to the root cause of what is tiggering your acne, it can also be a natural part of the surge in hormones that accompanies puberty. In serious cases, don't despair – seek the advice of a medical professional trained in treating acne.

ACNE AND 5 ALPHA REDUCTASE INHIBITORS

If you are looking to calm down the systems linked to DHT, try upping your intake of the following foods, which can slow the conversion of testosterone to DHT. This happens because of an enzyme called 5 alpha reductase. To recap, this is an enzyme that converts testosterone into dihydrotestosterone (DHT).

5 ALPHA REDUCTASE INHIBITORS:

Ground flaxseeds	Green tea
Turmeric	Onions
Coconut oil	Pumpkin seeds

WHAT ABOUT DAIRY?

Dairy products can be a fabulous source of protein, calcium, and iodine, but when it comes to hormone health, tread carefully with overconsumption. If you are experiencing skin issues such as acne, eczema, or psoriasis, have been diagnosed with PCOS or find that you are bloated after eating dairy, experiment with minimizing it and seeing how you feel. This could involve swapping cow's milk for a nut milk alternative. Look for nut milks with no more than two or three ingredients, such as almonds and spring water. Be cautious with oat milk, which can contain high levels of sugar. Consider reducing your cheese intake and sticking to a small amount of live yoghurt or kefir once or twice a week to see how you feel.

The overconsumption of dairy has the potential to be inflammatory, and it contains a hormone called insulin growth factor (IGF-1), which, at high doses, may mimic insulin. The A1 protein casein found in dairy is particularly inflammatory for the gut and negatively influences gastrointestinal transit times.

If you see an improvement after experimenting with minimizing dairy, stick to a little live yoghurt, cottage cheese, and parmesan occasionally, but switch out milk to a high-quality soy milk or nut milk. If you are supplementing your smoothies with protein powder, I also recommend sourcing a high-quality vegan protein powder over whey.

ULTRA-PROCESSED FOODS

Most food is processed in some way – the act of cooking is, itself, a process. However, there is a big difference between a home-cooked meal and the rise of ultra-processed foods, or UPFs, which are invading our supermarket shelves at an unprecedented rate. These are foods that undergo extensive levels of manufacturing processes, and are loaded with chemicals that could harm your health and your hormones' ability to function.

It's also worth avoiding foods with an unusually long shelf life, since this can be an indicator of the use of additional processes or preservatives. As a general rule, I'd recommend minimizing your intake of breakfast cereals, cheap ham, sausages or ultra-processed meats, bread, sweets, cakes, biscuits (cookies), and pre-made meals, to name a few. Ultra-processed foods are getting harder to spot, with many creeping into vegan aisles, nut milks, and children's snacks. These foods can drive inflammation and weight gain, playing havoc with your gut, blood lipids, and immune system. They also have the potential to drive diseases like type 2 diabetes and cancer. We cannot escape them entirely – I still keep fish fingers in my freezer and enjoy the occasional almond croissant. The positive power lies in what you do most of the time. Cooking food from scratch and knowing exactly what goes into your meals will help safeguard your health.

SPOTTING AND AVOIDING UPFS

The easiest way to avoid UPFs is to make meals from scratch wherever possible, using organic and high-quality ingredients.

Of course, not all foods can be made at home, and few of us have the time to bake our own bread every day. When you do need to buy something processed, always read the label, and ask yourself, "How much has this food has been faffed around with by humans or machines?" What is the "faff factor" involved in the production process? Look out for ingredients that you don't recognize. A few I would recommend avoiding include:

Aspartame

Emulsifiers like carboxymethylcellulose(466) and polysorbate-80(433)

Trans fat

Dipotassium phosphate, a synthetic acidity regulator

THE HALO EFFECT

Sometimes, labels can fool you into thinking you're making a healthy decision. Protein, for example, has become a popular way of selling food products, but remember that two eggs will provide you with as much protein as a protein bar. My cupboards contain plenty of processed foods – organic tofu, tempeh, parmesan – but these would not be classed as *ultra* processed. Just like running a marathon is not the same as running an *ultra* marathon.

As we'll learn in a moment, eating for hormonal health isn't a simple case of choosing the option with the lowest calories – a low-fat, flavoured yogurt might be lower in calories than "full fat" Greek yogurt, but it will likely be far more processed, and therefore could lead to a whole host of trouble for your endocrine system.

THE GREAT CALORIE DEBATE

Remember, you're eating food – not calories. Portion control and energy deficits can be necessary measures, but starving your body of the calories it needs will destroy your hormone balance.

Factors like gut health, metabolism, and insulin and cortisol levels all impact how we process food. Together, these factors determine something called caloric availability. If you continually try restricting your calorie intake, your body will adapt by lowering your basal metabolic rate to prevent starvation – a survival mechanism shaped by evolution. Underfeeding has been shown to trigger adaptive thermogenesis, where the body reduces energy expenditure and changes behaviour to encourage weight regain. This metabolic adaptation is more pronounced with dietary restriction than exercise, making sustained weight loss difficult.

NOT ALL CALORIES ARE EQUAL

A daily calorie allowance doesn't account for an individual's hormonal roadblocks, insulin levels, genetics, or gut microbiome – nor does it account for food's nutritional value. Forget all this, and you can forget long-term results.

Like the "sugar is sugar debate", you can't ignore calories as a metric. But for the sake of your hormones, you're better off looking at the ingredients in the food and how they might drive diet-induced inflammation – rather than just counting the calories.

Consider sweet potato. Are you eating it cooked? Are you eating it cooled after cooking? Are you eating it on an empty stomach? Are you eating it styled with protein, healthy fats, and an array of colourful vegetables? Depending on how you cook it and what you eat with it, the caloric availability and biochemical reaction to that same sweet potato could vary wildly, meaning that it could have a range of outcomes on your endocrine system. Five hundred calories of doughnuts will have a different impact than 500 calories of salmon styled with green leafy vegetables and chickpeas. If you make the wrong choices, your body will become stressed, inflamed, insulin-resistant, and nutrient-deficient, putting your hormones under enormous strain. Instead of focussing on metrics, look to eating food that creates a happier home for your hormones. Count your nutrients – not your hormones.

EATING FOR YOUR HORMONES
WHATEVER YOUR AGE

The first three pillars of the Positive Method have looked at different ways that nutritional choices can improve hormonal health. This guide details the smartest approach to nutrition depending on your body's needs.

LIFE STAGE	POTENTIAL CONCERNS	WHAT TO MAXIMIZE
PUBERTY	First period PMS Contraception Acne	Iron-rich foods Anti-inflammatory foods Zinc Vitamin A and E for skin
MENSTRUAL CYCLE	Irregular cycles PCOS PMDD Endometriosis	Vitamin D Prebiotics and probiotics Anti-inflammatory foods
PRECONCEPTION AND PREGNANCY	Infertility Miscarriage	Prebiotics and probiotics *Lactobacillus* for vaginal microbiome Vitamin D Antioxidants Omega-3 Folate Protein
POSTNATAL	Breastfeeding Post-natal nutrient depletion Low energy Postnatal depression	Omega-3 Iron-rich foods Magnesium Antioxidants B vitamins
PERIMENOPAUSE	Hot flushes Anxiety Weight fluctuations Mood changes Brain fog Menstrual changes	Phytoestrogens Protein
POSTMENOPAUSE	Bone health Muscle mass Weight fluctuations	Calcium Fibre

PILLAR THREE
EAT SMART
RECAP

o   Eat smart, not less.

o   Don't focus on calories alone –
consider the nutritional benefit of the
food as a whole.

o   Combine prebiotic and probiotic foods to
support a healthy gut microbiome.

o   Support your liver to optimally
clear hormones.

o   Reduce your intake of ultra-processed foods
and non-organic fruits and vegetables.

Pillar Four
Move More

Let's up the ante and discuss movement, muscle mass, and energy expenditure. You don't need me to preach the benefits of exercise – we all know that healthy movement improves mood, energy levels, sleep, and overall wellbeing. It also supports your hormones at every stage of the journey.

For teenagers, staying active can help regulate periods and menstrual symptoms, as well as supporting healthy bones for growth and development. During pregnancy, movement can ease hormonal symptoms like fatigue, while increasing blood flow through movement will help to reduce discomfort. For women going through the menopause, exercise is particularly helpful for managing weight changes and strengthening bones, reducing the risk of falls and fractures and helping you to feel stronger for longer. And at every single life stage, movement is brilliant for mental health, boosting endorphins and serotonin so you can better handle life's challenges.

One particular benefit of movement for hormonal changes is that it improves your muscle mass, safeguarding your skeletal mass index and lowering your risk of insulin resistance. Your skeletal muscle – the scaffolding for your skeleton – is not just there for locomotive function; it's a metabolic organ, and plays a central role in the body's energy and protein metabolism. The growing consensus is that your muscle mass is a gauge of health and can predict longevity.

Movement is closely linked to insulin and glucose metabolism. Skeletal muscle is a major target organ of insulin, where it first looks to store glucose. The more muscle you have, the better your insulin sensitivity will be, allowing for greater glucose uptake by skeletal muscles and enhancing the process. A healthy muscle mass means that you will function better as a metabolic machine and have more space for insulin to store glucose as glycogen before storing it as fat around your organs and middle. This means that you are going to feel more energized, as your body will be more efficient at regulating blood sugar levels.

The more robust your skeletal muscle, the stronger the scaffolding will be for your bones. This is especially important in later life, when bone density decreases. With the onset of menopause, skeletal muscle mass and strength also start to decline. Evidence shows that oestrogen-based HRT can significantly benefit skeletal muscle mass, strength, and protection from damage in older women.

MOVEMENT FOR EVERY LIFE STAGE

Healthy exercise is important at every life stage. Guidelines in the UK and US suggest that everyone should aim for at least 150 minutes or 2.5 hours of moderate to intense activity per week. Ideally, we should move for at least 10 minutes every day.

Aim to include a mixture of:

Cardio – This includes anything that raises your heart rate and has you breaking a sweat – think cycling or running.

Strength training – This means using exercise machines, free weights, or even your own body weight to build strength.

Low-impact exercise – This is gentle movement such as walking, yoga, and pilates, and benefits cardiovascular health as well as supporting strength training.

LET'S GO!

Maybe you struggle to fit in any exercise around your already busy daily routine, or perhaps you're a seasoned runner. Either way, it can be easy and enjoyable to create a routine that incorporates different types of exercise – including cardio, strength-training, and lower-intensity movement. Finding the right combination of movement for you is one of the most valuable things you can do for your hormones, longevity, and overall health.

Like many other millennials, I grew up in the days of fasted exercise and intense cardio. During my PCOS peak and in the lead-up to my stage 4 endometriosis flare-up, I remember training for the Great North Run, frequently running for long, unsafe distances in a fasted state. This was disastrous for my cortisol levels, but I was convinced it was the best way to train. Working out after an overnight fast is based on the theory that low glycogen levels cause your body to shift energy utilization away from carbohydrates, thereby allowing for more significant mobilization of stored fat for fuel in endurance exercise. But our ability to burn fat is not based on a minute-by-minute, hour-by-hour scenario – the composition of our bodies is based on healthy habits that can be implemented in the long term. These days, I know that energy (from food) is vital for exercise, and to build and maintain muscle in a healthy, sustainable way.

MOVEMENT AND NUTRITION

Moving in the morning is a great way to start the day. It is often more time-efficient as it's easier to squeeze in before your day gets going. It can also align with your hormones and body clock, since cortisol levels are naturally higher in the morning. Over-exerting yourself in the evenings has the potential to boost cortisol levels when they should be dropping, readying your body for melatonin and bedtime.

MOVEMENT AFTER EATING

The best way to support your body, regulate blood sugar, and harness the power of your hormones is to move and build muscle mass after eating. Your body then uses the nutrients provided and the glucose and insulin created in a positive way, aiding fat loss and skeletal muscle mass. Exercise helps to move glucose out of your blood and into your cells. It causes your muscles to contract – the only time in which your cells can absorb glucose for energy without relying on insulin. This helps your insulin stay reactive, allowing your cells to become more adept at using insulin and ultimately improving your insulin sensitivity.

Movement does not always have to be intense. Try building in a brisk 15- to 20-minute walk after breakfast, lunch, or dinner at least three days of the week. Of course, remember to first give yourself time to digest. Thirty minutes of brisk walking after meals has been shown to improve the glycaemic response after meals, but even 15 or 20 minutes

MOVING FOR YOUR HORMONES

Any form of moderate exercise is better than no exercise at all, but some forms of movement can be particularly beneficial during certain life stages, or while living with particular hormone-related health concerns.

LIFE STAGE OR CONCERN	MOVEMENT ADVICE	REASON
PUBERTY	Build bone strength and heart health through sports like netball, football (soccer), athletics, and dancing.	This is a period of rapid growth. Staying active can help you regulate periods, alleviate menstrual symptoms, and support bone development.
MENSTRUAL CYCLE	Work with your cycle and prioritize restorative, low-impact exercise during your period and when you experience PMS. Focus on higher-intensity training during ovulation and the follicular phase (days 6–14 of your cycle).	Movement can ease PMS thanks to mood-boosting endorphins, offering a natural way to manage symptoms. Adjusting exercise to your cycle can optimize workouts.
PCOS	Combine strength training with restorative exercise.	Strength training boosts insulin sensitivity by promoting muscle growth. Restorative movement helps lower cortisol levels.
HIGH STRESS AND BURNOUT	Combine restorative exercise with slowing down, incorporating long walks and yoga.	Slowing down with restorative movement can calm the nervous system.
PRECONCEPTION AND PREGNANCY	Explore restorative, pregnancy-safe yoga and pilates. Only continue with cardio and high-intensity training that your body is already accustomed to.	Gentle exercise during pregnancy can improve mood, reduce the risk of gestational diabetes, and promote faster recovery and overall wellbeing for both mother and baby.
POSTNATAL	Focus on pelvic floor exercises, gradually building from lower-impact to higher-impact exercise.	Pregnancy and delivery can weaken the pelvic floor, so it's important to gradually build up strength and allow your body time to heal before engaging in more intense activities.
PERIMENOPAUSE AND MENOPAUSE	Try functional strength training to help improve bone density and muscle mass, pilates for mobility, and yoga for flexibility.	Focus on muscle mass, bone density, and flexibility to reduce injury risk and supports health during menopause.
POST MENOPAUSE	Try weight-bearing exercise, brisk walks, and low-impact exercises like water aerobics for joint care.	Weight-bearing, low-impact exercise supports bone strength and muscle health, counteracting the effects of declining oestrogen.

can work wonders. It's a wonderful way of getting outside and enjoying a full spectrum of light on your face to reinforce your body clock (see Pillar Five on p.184). It supports and balances your blood sugar, and cultivates a positive mindset (see Pillar Six on p.195) by providing space to recharge.

MOVE FOR YOUR MOOD

Moving more is a surefire way of boosting your endorphin levels. When you exercise, you release feel-good endorphins (your painkiller hormone) that can improve your mood and sense of wellbeing. Studies show that exercise can improve mental health symptoms for depression and anxiety, as well as improve general resilience and frame of mind.

SEEKING BALANCE

I once subscribed to the mantra of "Go hard or go home", but this approach can be profoundly counterproductive for your hormones. Have you ever signed up for an intensive series of exercise classes in January, hoping to undo the indulgences of the party season? In the long run, these short-lived, frantic bursts of activity may not serve you. Overdoing it with high-intensity workouts on a regular basis can drive hormone dysfunction in women, and put pressure on your stress response via the HPA axis (see p.56).

Studies have shown that anabolic hormones – your growth hormones – are boosted after intense bouts of exercise. This makes sense, as "growth" is the basis of fitness. The results of a 2002 study looking into the hormonal responses to endurance and resistance exercise concluded that an acute bout of physical exercise can increase levels of oestradiol, testosterone, DHEA, and growth hormone in female subjects between the ages of 19 to 69 years. This rise in hormones builds muscle, boosts endurance and improves fitness. However, an influx of hormones must be balanced with adequate rest.

Endurance exercise comes with its risks – it has the potential to negatively impact your hormones and your body. Marathons and extreme competitions aren't formulated for hormone health. The American College of Sports Medicine (ACSM) uses the expression "female athlete triad" to describe the dysfunction that can arise from intense endurance exercise. This includes the loss of the menstrual cycle, osteoporosis, and, sadly, disordered eating.

Finding balance means ensuring that you pair endorphin-boosting cardio or strength-training with more restorative forms of exercise. Don't be afraid of slowing down your movement. If calming your nervous system is the priority, or you are feeling overwhelmed by anxiety or stress when approaching movement, slow things down – but still move. Instead of running, walk. Instead of dancing to fast-paced music, move to a slower beat. Instead of fast reps with weight training, slow down your reps or use lighter weights. Once your nervous system feels looked after, take things up a notch.

EXERCISE TO MAXIMIZE

We all know that exercise is important. It helps you to feel good, increase your energy levels and energy expenditure, improve your cardiovascular health, and build muscle mass, among so many other benefits. Find an exercise routine depending on what your body needs at that moment, and what feels good to you, without comparing your choices to anyone else's.

You're not alone if you find fitness overwhelming, unenjoyable, or downright scary. This is partly due to to additional barriers that women face when it comes to exercising. Data in the UK suggests that 48 per cent of women don't exercise because they feel "too unfit" (even though this even more reason to try it out!), while 45 per cent said that they felt self-conscious about their bodies and 40 per cent worried they were simply "not good enough".

The most important part of movement is enjoying it. If you're into your HIIT, mix it up with some restorative exercise like yoga. If it doesn't get your endorphins pumping, don't commit to a 5 am bootcamp session in a soggy park. Instead, try something you'll look forward to, whether that's a walk in nature or an at-home yoga session before bed. You may need to try a few different activities to see what sticks. What follows are a few ideas to get you started.

WALKING

Whether in nature or through the city, walking is one of the best ways to get moving, especially if you spend your days tied to a desk. Aim for a daily step count that works for you, whether that's 6,000 or 10,000. If your work is sedentary, try investing in a stand-up desk or even an under-desk walking treadmill to get those steps in. As discussed, taking a walk after meals is also a great way to balance your blood sugar and support your overall hormone balance.

STRENGTH TRAINING

We've already touched on the importance of supporting your skeletal muscle, and strength training is the best way to go about it. Weight training can be intimidating, but you don't need to be a bodybuilder to feel the benefits of lifting weights and building strength. The stronger you are physically, the better you can support your hormones and your body overall.

Begin by lifting something easy and accessible, like water bottles or tinned beans, before progressing to heavier free weights. There are plenty of instructional YouTube videos, but I'd also recommend attending a few classes or even having a session or two with a personal trainer. A professional can check your form and ensure you're getting the most out of your training.

Strength training offers you the possibility of progressing gradually, from light weights to heavier ones. The sense of reward is second-to-none!

CARDIO

Cardio can positively impact your hormones by boosting serotonin and supporting oestrogen metabolism. Regular cardio also enhances the growth of beneficial bacteria and short-chain fatty acids (SCFAs), improving your gut health and creating a happier environment for your hormones to thrive.

RUNNING

Running is a powerful form of cardio that strengthens the heart and improves circulation, reducing the risk of heart disease, stroke, and high blood pressure. I adore running – all that is required is putting on a pair of trainers (running shoes), getting some tunes on, and you're off.

Make sure that you have proper footwear, a supportive sports bra, and some reflective clothing. Many sports shops also offer a complementary service where they look at your gait to ensure you're running correctly, which can also be helpful if you're new to running. Apps like Couch to 5k, Strava, and Nike Run Club are also a great way to get motivated, as is finding a running buddy. Start slow, wear a decent SPF, and properly fuel your body.

Remember that every runner has to start somewhere, even if it's 30 seconds of jogging followed by a brisk, five-minute walk. A decent playlist also helps – I created one on Spotify called The Positive Method More More, if you need a bit of inspiration!

DANCING

From disco to ballroom and even just a boogie around the kitchen, this is one of my favourite pastimes. It boosts memory and offers plenty of mental health benefits. One study found dancing to be the most effective form of exercise for depression. Anyone who loves dancing will know precisely why this is true – the sense of freedom and joy is unbeatable. Let loose solo to your favourite music or try following a dance workout on YouTube. For added social benefits, seek out a local class or check out what's playing live.

CYCLING

Hopping on a bike has many of the same benefits of running – it's just gentler on the joints. This makes it a better option if you are pregnant, going through the menopause, or simply want to safeguard your bones. Stationary bikes in gyms can be especially helpful when pregnant, providing an added layer of safety. Many spin classes on stationary bikes involve upbeat music and coordinated movement, so you can enjoy the added benefits of improved mood and reduced anxiety.

REBOUNDING

This is just a fancy word for bouncing on a mini trampoline, but I am obsessed with it. Not only does rebounding feel like you are shaking off all the accumulated negative energy of the day, but science and NASA back it up as an amazing form of movement. It's great for pelvic floor strength, balance, coordination, lymphatic drainage, and bone strength, and has been hailed as a great exercise for postmenopausal women to improve women-specific health risk factors such as bone health and pelvic floor muscle function.

RESTORATIVE EXERCISE

When you're going through hormonal changes – whether that's progesterone spikes before menstruation or a peak in cortisol during a stressful period – restorative exercise can be extremely healing and balancing.

Regular restorative exercises including yoga and pilates improve insulin sensitivity by reducing stress and promoting efficient glucose metabolism. Yoga improves circulation, which can support the functioning of your thryoid gland. Pilates, meanwhile, is great for improving pelvic alignment and supporting your pelvic floor, so it's an excellent option for pregnant, postnatal, and menopausal women.

Remember – there are plenty of restorative exercises that are more fast paced. Dynamic yoga flows can be quick and sweaty, combining cardio with more restorative elements. Similarly, pilates, often combines strength-training elements, thanks to its focus on core strength and use of your bodyweight as well as free weights. Pay attention to how you're feeling, adapting your movement by upping the ante or slowing down the pace. Never be afraid to do your own thing in a group class – focus on yourself, not on what everyone else is doing!

PILLAR FOUR
MOVE MORE
RECAP

o It's never too late to start moving.

o Find movement that you love.

o Take small steps to improving
   your strength, fitness, or flexibility.

o Use movement to boost joy, release
   stress, and connect with your body.

o Always fuel your workouts, creating
   time for movement after eating.

o Build muscle mass and strength later
   in life to improve your insulin sensitivity
   and cardiovascular health.

o Slow down and rest when you need it.

Pillar Five
Sleep Better

Sleep is fundamental to your health, with your circadian rhythm acting as the beat to your hormonal drum – the 24-hour cycle in which your body functions. And this rhythm is only as good as the clues you give it. Now that you have learnt how to style your starches (Pillar One, see p.133) and boost your colour intake (Pillar Two, see p.137), give your sleep and hormonal heartbeat some love. When your sleep or body clock is disrupted, your hormones won't operate on schedule either.

CORTISOL AWAKENING RESPONSE

Cortisol (see p.56) is the prime example of how this disruption affects the body. If your cortisol awakening response is operating sub optimally, you might be feeling sluggish in the mornings and finding it hard to get out of bed. It could be a sign of stress, sleep deprivation, or even burnout. Your cortisol awakening response is how your body takes you from a state of sleep to a state of alert (see p.64).

At the other extreme, what if your cortisol is spiking abnormally high in the morning? These excessive elevations of cortisol levels could indicate anxiety, or that you're consuming too much caffeine either in that early-morning window or that you are ovulating (see p.49). During ovulation, your cortisol awakening response can be higher than at other times of the month. This may present as feeling hyper alert as soon as you wake.

Improve your rhythm, cortisol awakening response, and sleep quality by:

Reminding your body it's morning by getting daylight onto your face

Encouraging melatonin production in the evening

Having a morning and evening routine

Think of that hazy feeling after a long-haul flight, not knowing whether it's time for breakfast or bed – a dysfunctional body clock is like permanent jetlag for your hormones. When your hormones don't know what timezone you are in, they'll struggle to carry out the right functions in the right order. That's why it's essential to regularly remind your body of the time, using routine and light exposure.

WHY GOOD SLEEP MATTERS

When it comes to a good night's sleep, there is no one-size-fits-all. While you need more sleep throughout puberty, you might find yourself getting less of it at other points in your life, with work, newborns, and menopausal hot flushes. Sleep changes throughout your life, but don't panic – no matter what life stage you find yourself in, it's possible to work with your body and find ways to adapt.

The amount and quality of sleep we get can still affect our health. Melatonin, cortisol, adrenaline, oestrogen, testosterone, progesterone, leptin, and ghrelin all impact sleep. And your sleep can affect how your hormones function. Here are just a few aspects of sleep that can impact hormonal health in particular.

SLEEP AND ENERGY

We all know that a good night's sleep gives us energy for the day ahead. However, not only does a poor night's sleep leave us tired – studies also indicate that we burn less energy as a result. This in turn can have a negative impact on blood sugar and healthy weight management. Inconsistent sleep patterns can be particularly challenging for the body, with a strong correlation found between poor sleep associated with shift work, obesity rates, and type 2 diabetes.

SLEEP AND GLUCOSE REGULATION

Sleep has a major influence on the 24-hour cycle of your glucose levels. The poorer your sleep, the poorer your body will be at regulating glucose. A 2024 Zoe study found that going to sleep earlier and having a consistent bedtime helped regulate glucose levels, concluding that sleep significantly affects how well you can control your blood sugar levels the next morning.

185

Research suggests that your nocturnal glucose tolerance during sleep reaches its lowest point in the middle of the night. However, as the night progresses, insulin sensitivity slowly improves, likely due to the delayed impact of lowered cortisol levels that come with the onset of sleep. By morning, insulin sensitivity is at its highest.

This cycle holds true if you've had a good night's sleep but, without proper rest, your body will struggle to regulate glucose, losing track of its correct rhythm. This puts you at risk of insulin resistance and inflammation.

Shift workers, sleep-deprived new parents, or women going through the hormonal shift of menopause must therefore take care when it comes to blood sugar balance – your body is at a more sensitive life stage, and may not handle high levels of sugar quite as effectively.

If you work shifts, minimize your exposure to sunlight on your journey home to improve daytime sleep. Use blackout blinds, an eye mask, and a light box to enhance your sleep environment, prioritizing your sleep quality.

SLEEP AND HUNGER LEVELS

Have you ever felt hungrier after a lousy night's sleep? Acute sleep deprivation reduces levels of the satiety hormone leptin in our blood and increases concentrations of the hunger hormone ghrelin. Frequently disrupted sleep can drive excessive food consumption, as often when we are tired, we don't make the healthiest choices, reaching for quick fixes that may be ultra-processed or high in sugar.

YOUR LIFE STAGES AND SLEEP

With endocrine disorders like PCOS and hormonal shifts such as perimenopause, there will likely be sleep disturbances. Among women, the prevalence of sleep disorders seems to increase with age. Sleep disturbance is, in fact, a prime feature of the menopause, thanks to hot flushes, which frequently come at night.

Your menstrual cycle can impact your sleep even on a month-to-month basis. Poorer sleep has been associated with the premenstrual phase and menstruation, and is even more common in women with PMS or suffering from severe menstrual cramps. The link is likely due to the sharp rise in progesterone.

PREGNANCY AND SLEEP

Pregnancy can pose particular challenges for sleep. Soaring levels of progesterone and hCG make sleep disturbances, even insomnia, common. Take advantage of rapidly rising progesterone levels during the first trimester, which can make you feel unusually drowsy – listen to your body and prioritize rest; you do need more sleep when creating life. Conversely, progesterone also causes nocturnal sleep fragmentation and, in late pregnancy, rising oxytocin levels, which is the hormone responsible for normal uterine contractions that sometimes peak at night.

It's one of nature's more frustrating paradoxes: at a time when you need more sleep, your body has an even harder time getting it!

MOTHERHOOD AND SLEEP

One of the most eye-opening (excuse the pun) parts of motherhood was going through intense sleep deprivation. It's a powerful reminder of just how much sleep affects your wellbeing. Imagine, then, the impact on your hormones.

It can be frustrating knowing how important your eight hours of sleep are when your responsibilities prevent you from enjoying them. Motherhood is full-on, and the nights can be carnage. During pregnancy, the placenta ensures melatonin levels stay high, peaking in the third trimester. Studies suggest this is closely linked to melatonin's antioxidant and neuroprotective benefits for infants. After delivery, though, melatonin levels drop. In this phase, you need to support your body in producing melatonin.

To do this, focus on positive things you can control. When facing disrupted sleep due to children, pets, or loved ones in your care, shift your focus to quality – not quantity. You might not be able to control the amount of sleep you get, but you can definitely improve its quality. Use routine to repeatedly remind your body what time of day it is and encourage melatonin production in the evening. The more melatonin and less cortisol present, the easier your body will find going back to sleep after a disruption. You'll also benefit from melatonin's antioxidant properties. Even after a night of less sleep than you'd like, if you have a good morning routine, you can improve your cortisol awakening response.

RESETTING YOUR BODY CLOCK

Your master body clock sits in your hypothalamus – a biological structure governed by a small group of neurons called the suprachiasmatic nucleus (SCN) that are nestled deep in your brain and act as your body's coordination centre. This 24-hour cycle sets your sleep, waking, and hunger patterns, and is fundamental to your hormonal health via your cortisol awakening response.

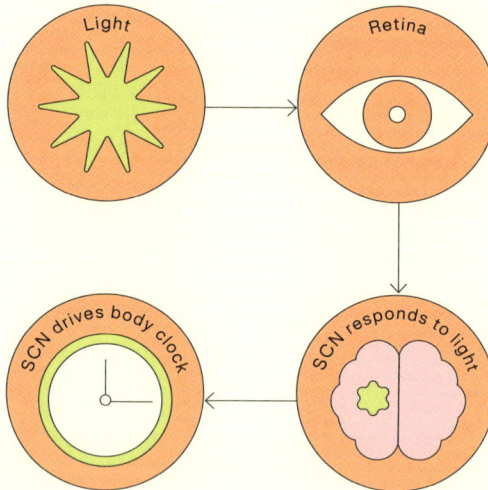

LIGHT AND BODY SYSTEMS
Light enters the retina and signals the SCN, which sets the body's internal clock.

Your body clock has cycles. If these cycles get mixed up, your body won't know what time it is, creating a downward spiral driving insulin resistance, inflammation, and other issues relating to your menstrual cycle. Your body clock's timing is only ever as accurate as the signals it receives. Perfecting these signals is key to creating a healthy environment in which your hormones can thrive.

WAKING UP

Your mornings have a knock-on effect on how well you will sleep at night. The first 30 to 45 minutes of your morning are precious, when your body transitions from a state of sleep to a state of awakening – a changing of the guard when your melatonin drops and your cortisol peaks. This transition sets the tone for your day, giving truth to this foundational bit of wisdom: a good night's sleep starts in the morning. Your morning routine can tell you a lot about your cortisol response. It's the perfect place to begin resetting your body clock.

Using the entire light spectrum is vital. Only natural daylight contains the whole spectrum, which you need to hit your retina in the morning. Once this light enters your retina, it stimulates the SCN, the body's master body clock in the brain, triggering a cascade of hormones to stimulate the peak in cortisol needed for a healthy awakening response.

DURING THE DAY

When it comes to getting a good night's sleep, it can seem like the odds are stacked against women – whether you're caring for a newborn, dealing with children waking up at all hours, working late, managing hormone dysfunction, or facing one of the many natural hormonal shifts that come throughout life. Research suggests that women are 40 per cent more likely to experience sleep problems than men.

We've already discussed the importance of preparing for a good night's sleep as soon as we wake: exposure to morning light is the most important factor for optimal pineal gland function.

Getting outside at any time of day is helpful; the amount and type of light you are exposed to throughout the day significantly impacts the maintenance of your circadian rhythm by regulating melatonin secretion. Essentially, the more you can remind your body that it's daytime during the day, the better prepared your body will be for sleep when nighttime comes.

Melatonin thrives in darkness, while cortisol rises in the first 35 minutes after waking. Our hormones thrive on routine – not unlike establishing a sleep pattern for a toddler or child. Establishing a good routine is key for your sleep pillar – waking up, eating, winding down, and going to bed at the same time every day. To support your hormonal health, try the following:

PREPARING FOR BED

From about 8 pm onwards, try limiting your exposure to blue light through devices like phones, tablets, and laptops. Blue light keeps melatonin at bay, making you more wakeful, and excessive exposure in the evening will confuse your body. Doomscrolling is therefore not only detrimental to your mental health; it will actively harm your rest. Blue-blocking glasses and screen protectors are helpful when you work late, but won't set you up for sleep mode.

Try not to eat or snack after 9 pm – your internal clock is regulated by the sun, as well as your eating patterns. The later you eat, the more work your digestion will also be doing when you should be falling asleep, ultimately impacting the quality of your sleep. See if you can enjoy a balanced, protein-rich dinner between 7–8 pm to ensure satiety through the evening. Then, if cravings come knocking, sip a calming herbal tea.

Find a space to charge your phone during the evenings, outside your bedroom. Leave it there at 8 pm, and don't check it again until after your morning cortisol awakening response.

SLEEP AND FOOD

Poor sleep can negatively influence your food choices, with sleep disturbances increasing ghrelin levels and driving the over-consumption of food. We're also learning that poor food choices can negatively impact sleep outcomes by affecting melatonin levels and its production from tryptophan.

Melatonin is a protein-based hormone, so if your sleep has been suffering, it can be helpful to have a diet rich in tryptophan, the amino acid from which melatonin (see p.75) and serotonin (see p.73) are derived. A colourful diet with lots of fruits, vegetables, legumes, and other sources of dietary tryptophan and melatonin has been shown to encourage better sleep.

THE SLEEP-ANXIETY CONNECTION

Let's face it: while there are multiple factors and hormonal shifts that affect our sleep, we often struggle to sleep because anxiety or worry keeps us awake. This might be because we're studying for exams or working in high-pressure jobs, or balancing parenting with caring responsibilities for elderly relatives.

It could help to try some pre-bedtime writing. Take a few minutes to note down whatever is worrying you. This activity has been proven to shorten the time it takes to fall asleep.

Remember, above all, to be kind to yourself to alleviate the pressures surrounding sleep. At important life moments the human body can also be extremely resilient. The more you can do to support your health holistically, the better you will counterbalance the impact of not getting enough high-quality sleep. Eating well, moving more, and seeking activities that actively combat stress will improve your sleep. This, in turn, will make you better equipped to adopt that holistically healthier lifestyle.

YOUR SLEEP CHECKLIST

A good night's sleep starts long before bedtime. Morning sunlight boosts cortisol, daytime activity keeps your rhythm steady, and an evening wind-down signals melatonin. By bedtime, a cool, calm space sets the stage for deep rest.

MORNING

- Get daylight onto your face when you wake up so your body knows it is morning, setting your internal clock for sleep to come later in the day.

- Get fresh air on your face, by going for a walk, stepping out your back door, or just popping your head out the window.

- Avoid screens for the first 30–45 minutes of the day – they can drive anxiety and stress by interfering with brain wave function.

- Boost your cortisol surge by introducing a routine of light stretches when you wake up.

- Stimulants like coffee can spike your cortisol – switch to drinking it after breakfast.

- Splash cold water onto your face to wake up, or, if you're feeling brave, try a burst of cold water in the shower.

- Try using a SAD lamp in the morning during the darker months of winter.

DAYTIME

- Throughout the day, as much as possible, allow for a full spectrum of light to remind your body it is daytime.

- Avoid caffeine from midday onwards, paying attention to your body's response; if you struggle with your sleep, try cutting it out entirely.

EVENING

- Limit blue light exposure after 8 pm to avoid disrupting melatonin production.

- Excessive screen time before bed harms health and rest, especially due to blue light's wakefulness effects.

- Blue-blocking glasses help at night but won't fully prepare your body for sleep.

- Avoid eating or snacking after 9 pm to prevent digestive disruption and improve sleep quality.

- Aim for a balanced, protein-rich dinner between 7–8 pm for evening satiety.

- If cravings arise, opt for calming herbal tea instead of eating late.

- Charge your phone outside the bedroom. Avoid checking it until 30 minutes after you wake up.

BEDTIME

- Check the time before bed to wind down and encourage your body to relax.

- Avoid intense exercise late at night, which raises cortisol levels and disrupts rest.

- Connect with loved ones, read, or take a calming bath to prepare for sleep.

- Dim lights and create a dark environment to boost melatonin production.

- Use a silk eye mask for a blackout effect – silk is kinder to the skin than cotton.

- Drink a bedtime tea with passionflower and chamomile to promote relaxation.

- Try meditation, white noise, or Epsom bath salts to calm your nervous system and sleep.

o   When life gets in the way of sleep, focus on quality, not quantity.

o   Hormones work best when your body clock is in sync, and quality sleep creates an environment in which they thrive.

o   Reset your body clock by getting outside in daylight.

o   Build a positive evening routine, with a wind-down incorporating evening tea, a bath, or breathwork.

o   Boost melatonin levels in the evening by dimming your lights and minimizing screen-time distractions after 8 pm.

o   Give your body the raw material – tryptophan – to make your sleep hormone melatonin by including foods rich in this amino acid.

Pillar Six
Live Positive

We only get one go at life, and it goes by fast. In this pillar, I want you to grab today by the horns, implementing positive actions to honour your nervous system.

Hormones and mood are profoundly interconnected. While hormones can affect your mood, high stress levels and negative emotions can create a hostile environment for your hormones, turning into a vicious cycle. Hormone dysfunction can leave you vulnerable to mood disorders, while PMS, pregnancy, postnatal depression, and the mood swings accompanying perimenopause and menopause are worsened by stress.

Here, we're going to learn how to mitigate this cycle. So, take a deep breath, unclench your jaw, and relax. Let's begin.

HORMONES AND STRESS

Life challenges our nervous systems before we even consider hormone balance. Add in the natural hormonal shifts experienced by women, as well as widespread endocrine disorders such as endometriosis, PCOS, PMS, and PMDD, and it is clear why levels of anxiety and depression are at an all-time high.

Not to put a dampener on our positive pillar, but we do need to cover some serious concerns. The statistics are alarming, and it's crucial we talk about them. Struggling with hormones can leave us vulnerable to low self-esteem, anxiety, and depression. That's why the positive tools in this book, especially in this pillar, are so important.

Women with PCOS are three times more likely to experience anxiety. Low progesterone and serotonin levels can drive anxiety, while PCOS symptoms can affect self-esteem and body image. Endometriosis also increases the risk of depression and anxiety which, frustratingly, can intensify the severity of pain experienced.

During perimenopause and menopause, the incidence of depression can double. This is thanks to symptoms that negatively impact quality of life and the decreasing levels of feel-good hormones. In the precious yet daunting postnatal phase, there is a risk of postpartum depression, a debilitating mental disorder. Additionally, post-traumatic stress disorder (PTSD) can occur at any point in life, dysregulating your HPA axis and increasing the risk of endocrine disorders.

Despite all of this, there are ways of taking control of your destiny and your genetic expression. Just as conditions can negatively manifest from life events, the severity of conditions can also be lessened through positive actions associated with diet and lifestyle. You cannot cure PCOS, for instance, but you can radically improve its expression and your symptoms.

Research shows that women are twice as likely as men to experience anxiety and depression. A growing body of literature links these mental states with fluctuations in sex hormones and their impact on the female brain. Thanks to the unique plasticity of the female brain, oestrogen plays a major role in determining its structure and function. A 2022 review concluded that the functional connectivity in the female brain is dynamic and shifts with fluctuating sex hormone levels, contributing to a higher risk of depression and anxiety.

By creating a happier, more stable home for your hormones, you can profoundly improve both your physical and mental wellbeing. Mental health struggles and hormonal shifts or imbalances are often connected to a nervous system trapped in "fight-or-flight" mode.

MANAGING STRESS

Stress has a physical dimension, primarily driven by the hormone cortisol. While hormones like cortisol are essential for the functions in your body, unmanaged stress can become a roadblock to optimal health and happiness. Supporting your nervous system is key for lasting results – neglecting it can limit the effectiveness of the other methods outlined in this book.

There's nothing worse than someone telling you to just "stop worrying" or advising you to "stress less". Spoiler alert: I do not have the secrets to removing your sources of stress. We all face challenging moments; they form an essential part of the human experience. But what happens to your hormonal health when you are regularly – or constantly – in a state of high stress? As a result, the body behaves as if it is under threat (see pp.99–108). This is a massive burden on your system, and a cascade of mechanisms can drive hormonal dysfunction in your body. Remember, we have not evolved to differentiate stress, whether its source is from working life, exams, divorce, financial worries, or motherhood. It has the same impact on your body and your hormones.

Stress can have profound implications, impacting everything from your weight to your reproductive health – several studies have underlined a correlation between infertility and high levels of cortisol.

Cortisol (as we learnt on p.56) is a master hormone that acts like a foghorn, amplifying the body's stress response.

WHEN OUT OF BALANCE, CORTISOL CAN:

Drive insulin resistance	Cause poor decision-making
Facilitate disease	Impair your sleep
Disrupt metabolism	Trap you in "fight-or-flight" mode
Spike your glucose	

THE ROOT OF THE PROBLEM

It might sound counterproductive, but let's look past your sources of stress. Whether you're facing challenges at home or at work, shift your attention towards changing the narrative for your nervous system. We may not be able to tackle the big stuff here, but we can intentionally invite little moments of joy.

IMMEDIATE ACTIONS

The goal is to lower your baseline cortisol. You can achieve this by working with your nervous system, reminding it on a regular basis that you are safe and not under threat, ultimately getting out of that state of fight or flight.

Instead of trying to solve issues that may be out of your control, work on creating frequent pockets of positivity. These could be as simple as a five-minute meditation or breathing exercise between errands or meetings. It could mean putting aside time to pamper yourself with a special treat or an indulgent night in. Invite more joy into your life with activities involving breathwork, play, self-love, creativity, rest, kindness, gratitude, and getting outside and into nature. Lean on people you love, and make time for laughter. Opportunities for human connection will boost your love and bonding hormone oxytocin – cortisol's kryptonite. Spending time with people you love and living fully in the present moment is just as important as eating your vegetables.

It's important to focus on the little things; otherwise, life can feel overwhelming. Multiple moments of positive action will add up to create a tapestry and form a feeling, one that reminds the body that it is not under threat. This rewrites the script for your nervous system and dampens your stress response.

PRIORITIZING YOURSELF

Women frequently find themselves in caregiving roles as daughters, mothers, sisters, and partners. As a result, we often place ourselves and our needs on the backburner. And our hormones sometimes bear the brunt of this pressure. Mothers, on average, report feeling higher levels of guilt than fathers, and for working mums, it can feel like you have to work as if you don't have children and have children as if you don't work. Alarmingly, alcohol consumption is on the rise for females in middle adulthood. A recent study looking into US alcohol consumption found that binge drinking and alcohol-related harms were increasing, primarily driven by women in their thirties and forties.

Meanwhile, time for wellness and mindfulness might feel out of our reach. Fitting in a self-care routine may seem laughable when the steam from a dishwasher is the closest thing to a facial you're getting. Does caregiving happen to the detriment of our stress levels? Are you finding yourself at the bottom of the pile?

It can feel uncomfortable, but whether you're 18 or 80, putting yourself first is not selfish – you may truly need it. Book into that yoga class. Spend some time alone. Say no to plans. Set boundaries. You cannot show up for everyone all of the time.

THE POSITIVE CHECKLIST CHALLENGE

For five days, try doing this simple exercise. In the morning, write down:

....

Three positive actions

....

One moment of gratitude

....

You may not realize it at first, but these positive actions will make your world brighter. Ask yourself, honestly, what is it that you love to do? Dig deep and reconnect with what makes you tick.

Some positive actions you could pursue might be creative, centred around relaxation, physical activity, or connection with nature. You might find it beneficial to focus on social connection or mental health, or simply activities that are entertaining or uplifting. Next, I will share some examples to get you started.

It's never too late to change direction and become the person you want to be. Sometimes, that means prioritizing yourself and stepping out of your comfort zone.

Positivity attracts positivity, and kindness has a ripple effect. Practising kindness can not only boost your oxytocin levels, but it can also be incredibly powerful for individuals with anxiety or depressive disorders. A recent study demonstrated that performing acts of kindness promoted social connection, a construct that is a key predictor of both wellbeing and recovery from anxiety and depressive disorders. Kindness doesn't have to cost a thing – smile at that stranger on your walk, hold the door open, compliment someone, ask how someone is doing, send that text, write that card.

This checklist is not meant to make you feel guilty about activities you no longer have time for. When life gets busy, self-care and hobbies can fall by the wayside. But now is the time for a change. Remember that you are reading this because you want optimal health, energy, and joy. So, let's commit! That will not happen independently – you need to invite this in. Determine what positive actions best serve you.

Start small. Reflect on what you most enjoyed from the challenge, then look forward. Decide which positive actions you want to make non-negotiable parts of your life. Incorporate them into existing activities.

POSITIVE ACTION CHECKLIST

By the end of the five days, you will have completed 15 activities that hopefully made you joyful. Repeat them the following week: this brings you to 30. The ultimate goal is to build up a toolkit of positive actions.

MENTAL HEALTH & SPIRITUALITY

If you're spiritually minded, connecting to the universe, a higher power, or whatever God you believe in can work wonders for the mind and soul.

EXAMPLES:

Try 10 minutes of breathwork

Meditate

Pray

SOCIAL CONNECTION

Connecting with loved ones boosts happiness, reduces stress, and improves wellbeing. Loneliness is as harmful as smoking 15 cigarettes per day. To feel the full benefits, be intentional and present, thereby boosting your oxytocin and serotonin levels.

EXAMPLES:

Tell someone you love them

Have a cuddle on the sofa

Set aside quality time for your loved ones

Donate to a food bank or charity shop

Write somebody a letter and post (mail) it to them

Plan a surprise for someone

Call your best friend

ENTERTAINMENT

Whatever your chosen form of entertainment, be intentional and present. You don't always need to be productive – sometimes, zoning out with your favourite show is enough.

EXAMPLES:

Curl up with a book or a magazine

Listen to a podcast

Watch a film

Dance to your favourite album

Pick an outfit that empowers you

We've covered the benefits of movement; now, combine it with nature. Studies show that connecting with nature generates joy and reduces anxiety and depression. Time outdoors is excellent for your nervous system and stress recovery.

EXAMPLES:

Take a walk in nature

Go for a cycle

Practise yoga

Plant something

CREATIVE

Creative pursuits help us enter a "flow" state, where we're fully absorbed and lose track of time – a meditative experience. Creativity isn't limited to art; it could mean arranging flowers, decorating, styling outfits, or even organizing your cupboards. Lean into your creativity, wherever it may be.

EXAMPLES:

Make a painting or doodle

Compile a photograph album

Start a vision board

Make someone a gift

Try a new craft, like knitting or sewing

Add colour with dopamine dressing

RELAXATION

Relaxation is about tending to your body, comforting yourself, and slowing down – no expensive treatments needed, just mindful self-care.

EXAMPLES:

Take a 20-minute bath

Take a luxurious nap

Do some restful stretches

Give yourself an at-home facial or manicure

Try out some facial and scalp massage techniques

Part of the reason I got my dog Twiggy was to make going for a walk non-negotiable, no matter the weather. Walking after my breakfast supports my blood glucose regulation, and the calming effect of being with a dog, spending time in nature, and enjoying exposure to the entire light spectrum can remind the body to relax and function optimally.

INCORPORATE POSITIVE ACTIONS INTO YOUR LIFE

You might wonder, where will I find the time to pick up painting? In a world where we can spend 40 minutes scrolling Netflix or social media, there's always space for small moments of joy to remind your nervous system that it's safe. This isn't about adding to your to-do list – it's about building more positive habits by incorporating them into your routine.

EXAMPLES:

If you commute, could you listen to a mindful podcast on the way to work?

In your morning shower, could you sing or say a few affirmations out loud, such as, "Today is going to be a great day", "The power is in my hands", or "I'm grateful for all that I have".

Try sitting around the table at dinner, phone-free, to ensure meals are quality time. And no matter the meal, I always light a candle at dinner – even if it's just eggs on toast.

WHERE IS THE COLOUR?

You might recognize this question from Pillar Two – but it goes beyond nutrition. Asking yourself, "Where is the colour?" in relation to your day-to-day life is about being more curious, creative, expressive, and open to new things.

Practising gratitude is a lovely way to start your day. This isn't just about expanding your cultural or positive action palette, but also recognizing some of the joy and colour that already exist in your life and that you might have sight of: your friends, your family, and the natural world around you.

Pick up a pen and make a little mental list for yourself now. Who and what are those cherished colourful glimmers in your life? Where are your creative outlets?

Ten minutes of breathwork before starting work for the day. Breathwork has done wonders for my hormone health. Your nervous system is intimately linked with your breath or respiratory rhythm. Box Breathing is an easy way to start. First, breathe in, counting slowly to four. Then, hold your breath for four seconds. Finally, slowly exhale through your mouth for four seconds. Repeat these steps for anything from five to 15 minutes. Focus on the air moving into and out of your lungs

Turn on some music in the kitchen and dance. I believe this is one of the best things you can do for your soul. Listening to music you love will make you smile more.

Dive into a fantastic story, whether by reading a book, listening to an audiobook, or watching a TV series or film you love. Fully absorb yourself in the present moment of a storyline without worrying about the past or the future. Even reality TV is great for this – there's no snobbery here.

Do something thoughtful. Kindness and human connection are proven ways of promoting resilience and happiness and reducing stress. I love to draw small illustrations, and during lockdown, I sent these illustrations to family and friends. This made me feel good, and it brought joy to others

Random acts of kindness can spread joy, whether smiling at a stranger, complimenting, or checking in on a friend – kindness is free and can enrich someone's day.

Try meditation, white noise, or Epsom bath salts to calm your nervous system and sleep.

Gratitude has been shown to have a positive impact on our lives. A glass-half-full mindset takes us out of reactive, high-stress mode and reminds us that everything is OK. Research has shown that optimism is linked to lower rates of depression and higher levels of wellbeing.

I don't want to push toxic positivity. Dismissing or invalidating negative emotions will not serve you. Terrible things happen in life, but remember that "this too shall pass". Seek the support you need, and be gentle on yourself when you need it. For the most part, if you can try to embrace a little more positivity, it will help you be more resilient.

One proverb I love tells us that holding onto negative energy is like holding onto a hot coal; in the end, the only one you burn is yourself. So, have a cry, scream, and shout, but remember that you have real power over what side of the bed you wake up on each morning.

THE POWER OF PLAY

As children, we are encouraged to play and be experimental. When life kicks in, though, these joyous and vital things can slip through our fingers as quickly as piles of laundry build up. Did you once love to dance? Did crochet ever appeal to you? Did you sing in a choir? Did you love to paint? What made you happy? Where was the colour and creativity? Sometimes, our creativity can be most stifled at the lowest point in our journeys. This is a pattern I often see with women in my clinic.

SEEK HELP WHEN YOU NEED IT

A little bit of stress is part of everyday life – but if you're suffering and feel like you have lost control, seek help. Reach out to a doctor or qualified professional. You are not alone, and there are many ways of getting support. Small acts of self-care are different from needing therapy or medication. If you've been feeling anxious or depressed daily for over two weeks, impacting your life or relationships, or have thoughts of self-harm, contact a doctor or professional. You're not alone, and support is available.

PILLAR SIX
LIVE POSITIVE
RECAP

o   Prioritize small moments of joy that
    snowball to create happiness, which
    will positively impact your body.

o   Take positive actions to signal safety
    to your nervous system and remind your
    body it's not under threat.

o   Ask yourself, where is the colour in your world?

o   Try the five-day positive checklist challenge,
    picking the actions you enjoy most.

o   Build a stress-relief toolkit with activities
    that genuinely make you happy.

o   Choose stress-relief methods that work
    for you; if silent meditation isn't your thing,
    try breathwork.

o   Maximize time with people who energize you.

o   Lower your cortisol levels by fostering
    calm through creativity, kindness, gratitude,
    and self-love – it's just as vital as eating
    nutritious food.

Conclusion

And that, my friends, is your toolkit for ensuring your hormones have the best possible environment to thrive – no matter what life stage you're at.

Over the course of this book, you'll have become aware of the many factors that can impact your hormone health. But while the causes are complex, the solutions don't have to be. The Positive Method enables you to cut through the noise, giving you everyday options and simple suggestions to help you thrive. You might not always be able to embrace every pillar, but each of these tools is here to support you whenever you need it. Together, these small changes build up to make a lasting difference. And the best time to begin is now.

READ THE ROOM

My biggest piece of advice for taking control of your health is to read the room. When we're about to tell a story or a joke, or to speak up in a meeting, we take a look around and ask ourselves: What does the room need right now? What is the room telling me?

This applies to your health, too. Ask yourself: What is my body telling me? What do I need right now? Reading the room is about listening to yourself. Choose the tools that best serve you at that moment. Trust yourself, and trust your process.

You might be going through a particularly challenging time at work or with your studies. Reading the room could mean supporting your mental clarity and productivity by seeking to balance your blood sugar, using the tools outlined in Pillar One.

Perhaps you're undergoing a major upheaval in your life. You might be dealing with a newly empty nest, separation from your partner, or a loss. You might find it beneficial to regulate your nervous system by incorporating gentle, uplifting movement into your day, as we learnt in Pillar Four.

The Positive Method is no quick fix. Still, it's absolutely possible to see positive results after giving each pillar just two weeks of focus. Eventually, that will add up to three months. It's incredible what you can achieve for your hormones in this time.

Remember that there may be other health factors at play, such as diagnosed hormone conditions, surgery or medication. But depending on your symptoms, you should see results like improved energy, mental clarity, reduced bloating, and fewer cravings for sweets and refined foods in a matter of weeks. Just be patient with yourself – shouting at a flower won't make it bloom any faster. Honour your progress, wherever you are in your journey.

LET GO OF SHAME

You're here, reading this book, because you care about your health – nurturing an insulin-sensitive, nutrient-rich, gut-happy, strong, and calm body. The six pillars of the Positive Method are your ticket there, and they will help you to tackle whatever life throws at you. But life is also about growth, and no journey is linear. You are human, and it is natural that your focus will come and go.

If you are familiar with the shame that can accompany wellness culture, I ask you to leave it behind; it will not serve you. Wellness shouldn't make you feel like you're living two separate lives based on your behaviour. You're not "good" or "bad". You simply are. Telling yourself that something is off-limits will only make it more tempting. Shame breeds rebellion. We are never simply "unhealthy" or "healthy", and shattering this misconception is key to creating a better hormonal environment. Do not put your wellness on an unattainable pedestal.

THE PUNISHMENT OF PERFECTIONISM

Shame stems from perfectionism. Of course, consistency is key to good health, and positive change takes discipline, motivation, and accountability. Living a healthy life requires commitment. All this is true – but striving for 100 per cent perfection is an impossible goal.

When we feel like we've failed, it can trigger shame, which fuels anxiety, stress, and ultimately hormone dysfunction. New research shows that shame and self-criticism can negatively impact health by increasing the production of cortisol – the very thing we aim to manage. A study looking into cortisol levels and self-preservation proposed that threats to the "social self" can elicit shame, which, in turn, activates the hypothalamic-pituitary adrenal (HPA) axis. Judging ourselves based on progress or appearance also triggers stress, which contributes to hormonal imbalances and worsens mental health.

Guilt and shame come in many forms – whether it's following a punishing fad diet, comparing your life to social media, feeling "hangxiety" after a night out, struggling with parental guilt, overworking, or feeling you're not doing enough. It's a devilish mix of unrealistic standards, a vague sense of failure, and people-pleasing at your own expense. But you can't do everything, and you certainly can't please everyone. Striving for perfection only leads to feelings of failure.

OVERCOMING SHAME

We all recognize how horrible shame can feel. I've felt shame around my weight, my irregular periods, and when my fertility came into question. Overcoming shame has probably been the most momentous part of my hormone journey, but it doesn't happen overnight. It comes from regularly and consciously reminding ourselves that we have absolutely nothing to be ashamed of.

Counteract any feelings of guilt or shame by choosing not to sweat the small stuff. Maybe you need that big night out with the girls. Maybe spin class can wait. Maybe you need a break from revising. Maybe, for one night, you can't stick to your regular sleep schedule. Maybe during a hectic day, in between tending to elderly parents or collecting kids from school, you only have time to eat a few ultra-processed snacks. Life gets in the way sometimes, and that's OK.

If things don't go to plan, it doesn't mean you've failed. So long as you stick to healthy habits most of the time, you won't undo all your good work by pulling the occasional late night or skipping out on healthy movement for a few days. In fact, by having followed the Positive Method at all, your hormones will be far better equipped to deal with life's hiccups. From years of clinical work, I've learned that bumps in the road often precede the greatest periods of growth.

The fastest way to reach your health goals is slowly and steadily. Setting realistic expectations for yourself will help you to release any negative emotions and move forward in your journey with balance and acceptance.

DUST YOURSELF OFF

When we slip up, it can feel like all our good work has been undone, and we're back to square one. But it's key, at moments like these, to move on and try again. Think of bumps in the road as stepping stones in your success story. These learning moments are a pivot point to dust yourself off and dive back into the pillars.

If you skip your morning run one day, don't write yourself off for the rest of the week. Simply plan another run into your schedule for tomorrow, and commit to some other activities that can bring positivity and movement back into your life. If you start your day with an unbalanced meal, make a great choice for the next. Style your starches with a diverse rainbow bowl for lunch, and have a protein-rich dinner with lots of colour.

Say, for example, you're in the middle of a particularly stressful period and you don't have time to pick up ingredients, so you end up ordering a takeaway. This one moment won't undo all of your hard work. Next time, consider booking an online food delivery, or having some rainbow-coloured meals ready in the freezer. Reflect on what might help you next time, and then move forward.

STAYING FOCUSED

If your focus starts to wane, take yourself back to your *why*. Revisit your goals and your success story, as we did on pp.122–123, and why you are doing this in the first place.

When I find my focus dwindling, I bypass feelings of shame or guilt by looking forward and writing down my success story. As extra motivation, I sometimes get a fresh notebook or write notes to myself on my office pinboard. Getting into the right headspace and finding your motivation is vital for achieving results.

After revisiting your *why*, writing it down or even saying it aloud, go back to the very first pillar, Pillar One on p.125. Spend the week focusing on simply having a great breakfast, without any pressure to achieve anything else for seven days. Once you've got breakfast nailed, look ahead to start incorporating the next five pillars.

YOUR JOURNEY

Think of every slip up as just a "dot" along your journey. A few unhealthy decisions here and there won't hurt – we learn and move on. It's only if these dots start to connect and paint a picture that they may pull your body towards inflammation and stress. Be mindful of how often these dots appear. We can't do right by our hormones if we lose sight of what we're doing the majority of the time. If your dots start to add up, there will be negative consequences.

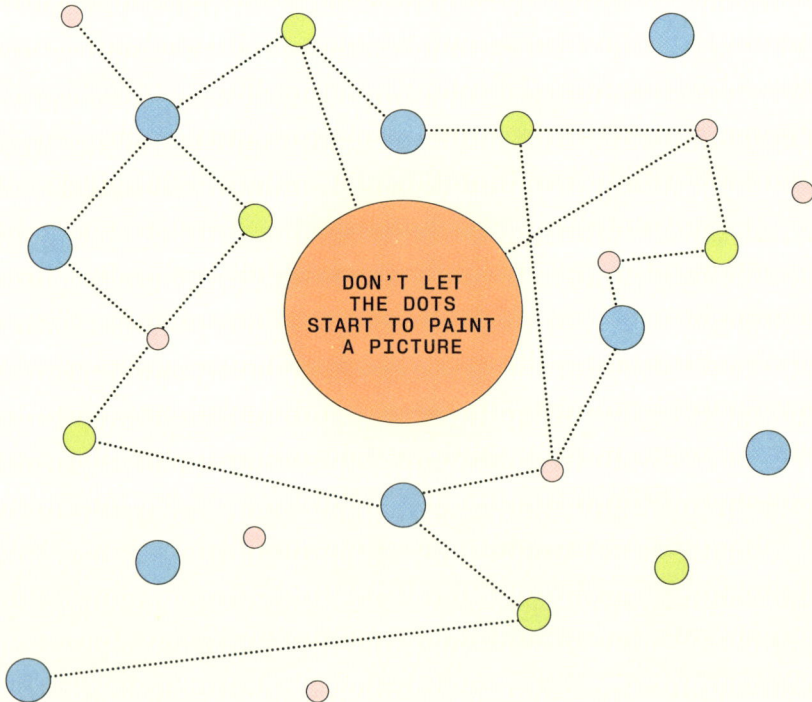

DON'T LET
THE DOTS
START TO PAINT
A PICTURE

Picture your future success and, at each crossroads, ask yourself: *is this choice moving me closer to my goals?* If that choice does not move you closer to your goals, you have the power to choose differently. Remember, you can't fail while undertaking the Positive Method. There is no such thing as failure if you try. Forgive any hiccups along your journey and keep looking forward, working to create a happier home for your hormones. Keep doing your best for your hormones, and your hormones will do their best for you.

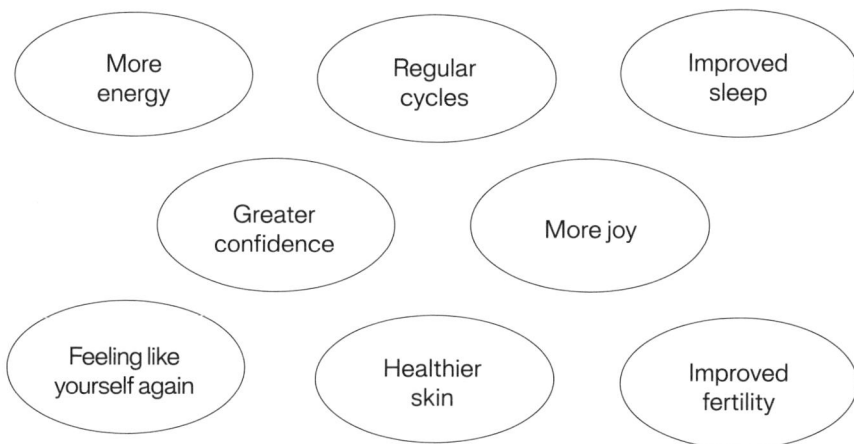

More
energy

Regular
cycles

Improved
sleep

Greater
confidence

More joy

Feeling like
yourself again

Healthier
skin

Improved
fertility

YOU'RE IN CONTROL

You hold the power. You make the choices that shape your health. You are here because you want positive change for your health, hormones, energy, and quality of life.

Remind yourself that you are building on everything you have learned in the Positive Method, and being as consistent as you can. You are balancing your blood sugar, eating colourful, eating smart, sleeping better, moving more, and living more positively.

Glossary

ANDROGEN
Any sex hormone that has "masculinising" effects, such as testosterone.

ANTIOXIDANTS
A substance that protects cells from damage by mopping up and neutralising free radicals.

CHOLESTEROL
The main substrate for sex and steroid hormone biosynthesis, meaning that it is the raw material for your steroid hormones.

DOPAMINE
The 'feel good' neurotransmitter. It plays a significant role in both movement and memory, and feelings of pleasure and reward.

ENDOMETRIOSIS
An oestrogen-dominant inflammatory condition that occurs when tissue similar to the lining of the uterus grows outside of the uterus, forming painful and inflamed lesions.

ENDOCRINE SYSTEM
A network of glands that produce hormones, regulating metabolism, growth, reproduction, mood, and overall homeostasis.

ESTROBOLOME
A collection of gut bacteria that regulates, circulates, and breaks down oestrogen, playing a crucial role in its clearance and balance within the body.

FREE RADICALS
Unstable molecules with unpaired electrons, generated by food, exercise, or toxins. They can cause oxidative stress.

HORMONES
Chemical messengers that travel around the body, regulating physiology and behaviour.

HYPOTHYROIDISM
An underactive thyroid gland, meaning that the thyroid does not produce enough hormones.

MICROBIOME
A microbiome is a community of microorganisms, including bacteria, fungi, viruses, and other microbes, living in a specific environment, influencing health and ecological functions.

MENOPAUSE
The cessation of menstruation (literally, the last period), marking the end of a woman's reproductive years.

METABOLIC SYNDROME
A collective term for health issues that put you at greater risk of type 2 diabetes or conditions that affect your heart or blood vessels. These include insulin resistance, cardiovascular disease, high blood pressure, and non-alcoholic fatty liver disease.

MITOCHONDRIA
Cellular powerhouses that convert glucose into ATP, providing energy for survival, function, and overall metabolic health.

PCOS
An endocrine disorder driven by an imbalance of hormones, typically producing excessive amounts of testosterone, cortisol, and insulin.

PERIMENOPAUSE
The transitional phase before menopause, when ovaries gradually become less active. There can be a rollercoaster of hormonal changes as sex hormones start to decline, with symptoms such as irregular periods, hot flushes, and mood changes.

PREMENSTRUAL DYSPHORIC DISORDER (PMDD)
A life-disrupting mood disorder, sharing some symptoms with PMS but operating at a much greater intensity. It is linked to fluctuations in progesterone, allopregnanolone, oestrogen, testosterone, and neurotransmitters like serotonin, GABA, and glutamate.

PREGNENOLONE
A precursor steroid hormone synthesised from cholesterol.

PUBERTY
The transitional stage during which a child matures into an adult. In girls, this is marked by physical changes like the development of secondary sexual characteristics including breast development, hip widening, and pubic hair growth, and the start of menstruation.

NEUROTRANSMITTER
A chemical messenger that carries signals between nerve cells, muscles, and glands.

ULTRA-PROCESSED FOODS (UPFS)
Foods which have undergone extensive processing and are packed with chemicals that may negatively impact your health and hormone function.

Resources

ONLINE RESOURCES & ORGANISATIONS

Bloody Good Period
www.bloodygoodperiod.com

Endometriosis UK
www.endometriosis-uk.org

Endometriosis Association
www.endometriosisassn.org

The Eve Appeal
eveappeal.org.uk

EWG's Shopper's Guide to Pesticides in Produce
www.ewg.org/foodnews

Lady Garden Foundation
www.ladygardenfoundation.com

The Menopause Society
www.menopause.org

Mind
www.mind.org.uk

PCOS Awareness Association
www.pcosaa.org

APPS

Calm
Mediation and sleep stories

Headspace
Meditation

Moody Month
Wellbeing for women, tailored to your cycle

Open
Breathwork exercises

Think Dirty
Educates users on potential toxins in household, personal care and beauty products

BOOKS - WOMEN'S HEALTH

Beyond the Pill
Dr. Jolene Brighten

The Fifth Vital Sign
Lisa Hendrickson-Jack

Hormone Repair Manual
Lara Briden ND

PCOS SOS
Felice Gersh MD with Alexis Perella

The Perimenopause Solution
Dr Shahzadi Harper and Emma Bardwell

Period Power
Maisie Hill

Real Food for Pregnancy
Lily Nicholas

The Science of Menopause
Dr Philippa Kaye

Wild Power
Alexandra Pope and Sjanie Hugo Wurlitzer

WomanCode
Alisa Vitti

BOOKS - PERSONAL DEVELOPMENT

How Emotions Are Made
Lisa Feldman Barrett

The Let Them Theory
Mel Robbins

Manifest
Roxie Nafousi

Smarter
Emily Austen

SUPPORT FROM THE AUTHOR

The Positive Method Club
www.thepositivemethodclub.com

The Positive Method Club is a private, algorithm-free community for you to connect with other women and feel inspired; a safe space to encourage, educate and empower you to feel your best. Enjoy meal plans, workbooks, recipes, live calls, resets and challenges, breathwork, the app, build your own profile and access to The 6 Pillar Positive Method course. Join a flourishing community of women alongside the expert guidance of Hannah.

One-to-one with Hannah Alderson
www.HannahAlderson.com

Experience bespoke one-to-one support and exclusive access to Hannah on a professional and personal level. Embrace a new lifestyle, gain an education into your hormonal health and nutrition, transform your relationship with food, and learn how to eat and live well for the rest of your life. This is perfect for those looking for an immersive, educational and life changing journey.

Clinical specialisms include PCOS, weight loss, fertility & IVF support, perimenopause/menopause, Eedometriosis, PMS, thyroid, acne, rosacea, and eczema.

Book your discovery call today via email: hello@hannahalderson.com

A concise version of this book's bibliography can be found below. For a full bibliography, including web links to articles available online, please go to: www.dk.com/hormones-biblio

THE LANDSCAPE OF
CHANGING HORMONES

14–19 Herman-Giddens et al. (1997). 'Secondary sexual characteristics and menses in young girls seen in office practice: a study from the Pediatric Research in Office Settings network'. Pediatrics, 99(4), 505–512. • Levine, H. et al. (2017). 'Temporal trends in sperm count: A systematic review and meta-regression analysis'. Human Reproduction Update, 23(6), 646–659. • Research Live. (2023, February 10). Report shows influence of social media for healthcare information. Research Live. • Department of Health and Social Care. (2022, July 20). Women's health strategy for England. GOV.UK. • York Health Economics Consortium. (2023). Women's priorities for women's health: A focus group study. University of York. • University of York. (2024, March 6). Research highlights delay in endometriosis diagnosis. University of York News. • Hearn, J. H. et al (2024). A COM-B and Theoretical Domains Framework. 'Mapping of the Barriers and Facilitators to Effective Communication and Help-Seeking Among People With, or Seeking a Diagnosis Of, Endometriosis'. Journal of Health Communication, 29(3), 174–186. • Carrot Fertility. (2024). Menopause in the Workplace 2024. • Hologic Global Women's Health Index. (2024). Year 3 Global Report. • Baird, D. T. et al (1999). 'Fertility and ageing'. Human Reproduction Update, 5(5), 482–486. • Swan, S. H. and Colino, S. (2023). 'Declining sperm counts: A global health concern'. In Advances in Reproductive Sciences (pp. 345–360). Springer. • Institute for Health Metrics and Evaluation. (2019). 'Dramatic declines in global fertility rates set to transform the population'.

THE HOUSE OF HORMONES

22–25 Murtagh, D. and Greenwood, M. (2010). 'The unethical use of BMI in contemporary general practice'. Postgraduate Medical Journal, 86(1012), 429–430.
28–31 Sawada, Y. et al (2021). 'Omega 3 fatty acid and skin diseases'. Frontiers in immunology, 11, 623052.
32–41 Brinton, R. D. et al (2015). 'Perimenopause as a neurological transition state'. Nature reviews endocrinology, 11(7), 393–405. • Yu, Z. et al (2022). 'Level of Estrogen in Females—the different impacts at different life stages'. Journal of Personalized Medicine, 12(12), 1995. • Yan, H. et al (2019). 'Estrogen improves insulin sensitivity and suppresses gluconeogenesis via the transcription factor Foxo1'. Diabetes, 68(2), 291–304. • Gu, W. (2022). 'Healthy long-lived human beings—Working on life stages to break the limitation of human lifespans'. Biology, 11(5), 656. • Hashemi, L et al (2024). 'Gender-Affirming hormone treatment and metabolic syndrome among transgender veterans'. JAMA Network Open, 7(7), e2419696–e2419696.
42–46 Kim, C. H. (2015). 'A functional relay from progesterone to vitamin D in the immune system'. DNA and Cell Biology, 34(6), 379–382. • Stefaniak, M. et al (2023). 'Progesterone and its metabolites play a beneficial role in affect regulation in the female brain'. Pharmaceuticals, 16(4), 520. • Meltzer-Brody, S. et al. (2018). 'Brexanolone injection in post-partum depression: two multicentre, double-blind, randomised, placebo-controlled, phase 3 trials'. The Lancet, 392 (10152), 1058–1070. • MacLean, J. A. et al (2022). 'Progesterone actions and resistance in gynecological disorders'. Cells, 11(4), 647.
47–51 Mei, M. et al (2022). 'Does scent attractiveness reveal women's ovulatory timing? Evidence from signal detection analyses and endocrine predictors of odour attractiveness'. Proceedings of the Royal Society B, 289(1970), 20220026.
52–55 Simitsidellis, I. et al (2018). 'Androgens and endometrium: new insights and new targets'. Molecular and cellular endo-crinology, 465, 48–60. • Davis, S. R. and Tran, J. (2001). 'Testosterone influences libido and well being in women'. Trends in Endocrinology & Metabolism, 12(1), 33–37.
56–65 Hewagalamulage, S. D. et al (2016). 'Stress, cortisol, and obesity: a role for cortisol responsiveness in identifying individuals prone to obesity'. Domestic animal endocrinology, 56, S112–S120. • Kuras, Y. I. et al (2017). 'Blunted diurnal cortisol activity in healthy adults with childhood adversity'. Frontiers in human neuroscience, 11, 574. • Hannibal, K. E.et al (2014). 'Chronic stress, cortisol dysfunction, and pain: a psychoneuroendocrine rationale for stress management in pain rehabilitation'. Physical therapy, 94(12), 1816–1825. • Smith, Allison, ND (2023). 'Assessing Chronic Fatigue with the Cortisol Awakening Response'. Precision Analytical Inc.
66–70 Straub, R. H. (2014). 'Interaction of the endocrine system with inflammation: a function of energy and volume regulation'. Arthritis research & therapy, 16, 1–15. • Ding, H. et al (2021). 'Resistance to the insulin and elevated level of androgen: A major cause of polycystic ovary syndrome'. Frontiers in endocrinology, 12, 741764. • De Bois, Maxime et al (2020). GLYFE: Review and Benchmark of Personalized Glucose Predictive Models in Type-1 Diabetes.
73–74 Yabut, J. M et al (2019). 'Emerging roles for serotonin in regulating metabolism: new implications for an ancient molecule'. Endocrine reviews, 40(4), 1092–1107. • Musial, N. et al (2021). 'Perimenopause and First-Onset Mood Disorders: A Closer Look'. Focus, 19(3), 330–337. • Bromberger, J. T. et al (2011). 'Mood and menopause: findings from the Study of Women's Health Across the Nation (SWAN) over 10 years'. Obstetrics and Gynecology Clinics, 38(3), 609–625.
78 Cera, N. et al (2024). 'The Role of Oxytocin in Polycystic Ovary Syndrome: A Systematic Review'. Current Issues in Molecular Biology, 46(6), 5223–5241. • Liu, N. et al (2022). 'Oxytocin in women's health and disease'. Frontiers in endocrinology, 13, 786271.
80–83 Turcu, A. F. et al (2015). 'Adrenal steroidogenesis and congenital adrenal hyperplasia'. Endocrinology and Metabolism Clinics, 44(2), 275–296.
84–86 Wu, C. Wei, K. et al (2017). '5α-reductase activity in women with polycystic ovary syndrome: a systematic review and meta-analysis'. Reproductive Biology and Endocrinology, 15, 1–9. • Zhang, Q. et al (2010). 'Circulating mitochondrial DAMPs cause inflammatory responses to injury'. Nature, 464(7285), 104–107.
87–91 Góralczyk-Bińkowska, A. et al (2022). 'The microbiota–gut–brain Axis in psychiatric disorders'. International journal of molecular sciences, 23(19), 11245. • Sun, L. J.et al (2020). 'Gut hormones in microbiota-gut-brain cross-talk'. Chinese medical journal, 133(7), 826–833. • He, S. et al (2021). 'The gut microbiome and sex hormone-related diseases'. Frontiers in microbiology, 12, 711137. • Filippone, A. et al. (2023). 'Endocrine disruptors in food, estrobolome and breast cancer'.

Journal of Clinical Medicine, 12(9), 3158. ▪ Lindheim, L. et al. (2017). 'Alterations in gut microbiome composition and barrier function are associated with reproductive and metabolic defects in women with polycystic ovary syndrome (PCOS): a pilot study'. PloS one, 12(1), e0168390. ▪ Pai, A. H. Y. et al. (2023). 'Gut Microbiome–Estrobolome Profile in Reproductive-Age Women with Endometriosis'. International Journal of Molecular Sciences, 24(22), 16301. ▪ Kwa, M. et al. (2016). 'The intestinal microbiome and estrogen receptor–positive female breast cancer'. Journal of the National Cancer Institute, 108(8), djw029. ▪ Hu, S. et al (2023). 'Gut microbial beta-glucuronidase: a vital regulator in female estrogen metabolism'. Gut Microbes, 15(1), 2236749.

92–93 Brennan, C. et al. (2024). 'Harnessing the power within: engineering the microbiome for enhanced gynecologic health'. Reproduction and Fertility, 5(2). ▪ Gliniewicz, K. et al. (2019). 'Comparison of the vaginal microbiomes of premenopausal and postmenopausal women'. Frontiers in microbiology, 10, 193. ▪ Park, M. G. et al (2023). 'Menopausal changes in the Microbiome—a review focused on the genitourinary Microbiome'. Diagnostics, 13(6), 1193. ▪ Grewal K et al. Chromosomally normal miscarriage is associated with vaginal dysbiosis and local inflammation. BMC Med. 2022 Jan 28;20(1):38. ▪ Vitale SG et al. The Role of Genital Tract Microbiome in Fertility: A Systematic Review. Int J Mol Sci. 2021 Dec 24;23(1):180. ▪ Bradford LL et al. The vaginal mycobiome: A contemporary perspective on fungi in women's health and diseases. Virulence. 2017 Apr 3;8(3):342–351. ▪ Park MG et al. Menopausal Changes in the Microbiome-A Review Focused on the Genitourinary Microbiome. Diagnostics (Basel). 2023 Mar 21;13(6):1193. ▪ Hillier SL et al. Vaginal microflora in postmenopausal women who have not received estrogen replacement therapy. Clin Infect Dis. 1997 Sep;25 Suppl 2:S123–6. ▪ Kim DS et al. Urinary Tract Infection and Microbiome. Diagnostics (Basel). 2023 May 31;13(11):1921.

99–108 Xing, Z. et al (2022). 'Association of age at menopause with type 2 diabetes mellitus in postmenopausal women in the United States: National Health and Nutrition Examination Survey 2011–2018'. Menopause Review/

Przegląd Menopauzalny, 21(4), 229–235. ▪ Yan, H. et al. (2019). 'Estrogen improves insulin sensitivity and suppresses gluconeogenesis via the transcription factor Foxo1'. Diabetes, 68(2), 291–304. ▪ Purwar, A. et al (2022). 'Insulin resistance in polycystic ovarian syndrome'. Cureus, 14(10). ▪ Chao, A. M. et al (2017). 'Stress, cortisol, and other appetite-related hormones: Prospective prediction of 6-month changes in food cravings and weight'. Obesity, 25(4), 713–720. ▪ Adam, T. C.et al (2007). 'Stress, eating and the reward system'. Physiology & behavior, 91(4), 449–458. ▪ Aboeldalyl, S. et al (2021). 'The role of chronic inflammation in polycystic ovarian syndrome— a systematic review and meta-analysis'. International journal of molecular sciences, 22(5), 2734.

109–15 Wang, X. et al (2021). 'Exploring the biological activity and mechanism of xenoestrogens and phytoestrogens in cancers: emerging methods and concepts'. International journal of molecular sciences, 22(16), 8798. ▪ Canivenc-Lavier, M. C. et al (2023). 'Phytoestrogens and health effects'. Nutrients, 15(2), 317. ▪ Ragnarsdóttir, O. et al (2024). 'Dermal bioavailability of perfluoroalkyl substances using in vitro 3D human skin equivalent models'. Environment International, 188, 108772. ▪ Loretz, L. J. et al. (2005). 'Exposure data for cosmetic products: lipstick, body lotion, and face cream'. Food and Chemical Toxicology, 43(2), 279–291. ▪ Marroquin, J. et al (2024). 'Chemicals in menstrual products: a systematic review'. BJOG: An International Journal of Obstetrics & Gynaecology, 131(5), 655–664.

THE POSITIVE METHOD

137–58 Hsu, M. C. et al (2018). 'Omega-3 polyunsaturated fatty acid supplementation in prevention and treatment of maternal depression: Putative mechanism and recommendation'. Journal of affective disorders, 238, 47–61. ▪ Winston, C. et al. (1999). 'Phytochemicals: health protective effects'. Canadian Journal of Dietetic Practice and Research, 60(2), 78. ▪ Thomson, R. L. et al (2012). 'Vitamin D in the aetiology and management of polycystic ovary syndrome'. Clinical endocrinology, 77(3), 343–350. ▪ Mei, Z. et al (2023). 'The role of vitamin D in menopausal women's health'. Frontiers in Physiology, 14, 1211896. ▪ Kim, K. et al (2020). 'Dietary intakes of vitamin B-2 (riboflavin), vitamin B-6, and vitamin B-12 and

ovarian cycle function among premenopausal women'. Journal of the Academy of Nutrition and Dietetics, 120(5), 885–892. ▪ Salve, J. et al (2019). 'Adaptogenic and anxiolytic effects of ashwagandha root extract in healthy adults: a double-blind, randomized, placebo-controlled clinical study'. Cureus, 11(12). ▪ Lee, S. et al. (2009). 'Adolescent and adult soy food intake and breast cancer risk: results from the Shanghai Women's Health Study'. The American journal of clinical nutrition, 89(6), 1920–1926. ▪ Messina, M. (2016). 'Impact of soy foods on the development of breast cancer and the prognosis of breast cancer patients'. Forschende Komplementärmedizin/ Research in Complementary Medicine, 23(2), 75–80. ▪ Dadkhah, H. et al (2016). 'Evaluating the effects of vitamin D and vitamin E supplement on premenstrual syndrome: A randomized, double-blind, controlled trial'. Iranian journal of nursing and midwifery research, 21(2), 159–164. ▪ Kamp, F. et al (2011). 'Effect of oral contraceptive use and zinc supplementation on zinc, iron and copper biochemical indices in young women'. e-SPEN, the European e-Journal of Clinical Nutrition and Metabolism, 6(6), e253–e258. ▪ Dording, C. M. et al. (2015). 'A Double-Blind Placebo-Controlled Trial of Maca Root as Treatment for Antidepressant-Induced Sexual Dysfunction in Women'. Evidence-Based Complementary and Alternative Medicine, 2015(1), 949036. ▪ Hamidpour, M. et al (2014). 'Chemistry, pharmacology, and medicinal property of sage (Salvia) to prevent and cure illnesses such as obesity, diabetes, depression, dementia, lupus, autism, heart disease, and cancer'. Journal of traditional and complementary medicine, 4(2), 82–88. ▪ Salve, J. et al (2019). 'Adaptogenic and anxiolytic effects of ashwagandha root extract in healthy adults: a double-blind, randomized, placebo-controlled clinical study'. Cureus, 11(12). ▪ Schellenberg, R. (2001). 'Treatment for the premenstrual syndrome with agnus castus fruit extract: prospective, randomised, placebo controlled study'. BMJ, 322(7279), 134–137.

159–73 Blanco-Pérez, F. et al (2021). 'The dietary fiber pectin: health benefits and potential for the treatment of allergies by modulation of gut microbiota'. Current allergy and asthma reports, 21, 1–19. ▪ Amabebe, E. et al (2020). 'Female gut and genital tract microbiota-induced crosstalk and differential effects of short-chain fatty acids on immune sequelae'. Frontiers in Immunology, 11, 2184. • Katz, E. et al (2018). 'Indole-3-carbinol: a plant hormone combatting cancer'. F1000 Research, 7. • Ağagündüz, D. et al (2022). 'Cruciferous vegetables and their bioactive metabolites: from prevention to novel therapies of colorectal cancer'. Evidence-Based Complementary and Alternative Medicine, 2022(1), 1534083. • Yan, L. et al (2023). 'Therapeutic potential of sulforaphane in liver diseases: a review'. Frontiers in Pharmacology, 14, 1256029. • DiNicolantonio, J. J. et al (2021). 'The importance of maintaining a low omega-6/omega-3 ratio for reducing the risk of autoimmune diseases, asthma, and allergies'. Missouri medicine, 118(5), 453. • Blasbalg, T. L. et al (2011). 'Changes in consumption of omega-3 and omega-6 fatty acids in the United States during the 20th century'. The American journal of clinical nutrition, 93(5), 950–962. • Mizawa, M. et al (2013). 'Stress evaluation in adult patients with atopic dermatitis using salivary cortisol'. BioMed research international, 2013(1), 138027. • Meštrović-Štefekov, J. et al (2018). 'Psychological stress in patients with atopic dermatitis'. Acta Dermatovenerologica Croatica, 26(4), 297–297. • Schiavone, F. E. (1983). 'Elevated free testosterone levels in women with acne'. Archives of dermatology, 119(10), 799–802. • Raghunath, R. S. et al (2015). 'The menstrual cycle and the skin'. Clinical and experimental dermatology, 40(2), 111–115. • Watling, C. Z. et al. (2021). 'Associations of circulating insulin-like growth factor-I with intake of dietary proteins and other macronutrients'. Clinical Nutrition, 40(7), 4685–4693. • Simpson, H. L. (1998). 'Insulin-like growth factor-I and diabetes. A review'. Growth Hormone & IGF Research, 8(2), 83–95. • Brooke-Taylor, S. et al (2017). 'Systematic review of the gastrointestinal effects of A1 compared with A2 α-casein'. Advances in nutrition, 8(5), 739–748. • Casanova, N. et al (2019). 'Metabolic adaptations

during negative energy balance and their potential impact on appetite and food intake'. Proceedings of the Nutrition Society, 78(3), 279–289.
174–83 Srikanthan, P. et al (2014). 'Muscle mass index as a predictor of longevity in older adults'. The American journal of medicine, 127(6), 547–553. • Haines, M. S. et al (2020). 'Association between muscle mass and insulin sensitivity independent of detrimental adipose depots in young adults with overweight/obesity'. International journal of obesity (2005), 44(9), 1851–1858. • Tiidus P. M. (2011). 'Benefits of estrogen replacement for skeletal muscle mass and function in post-menopausal females: evidence from human and animal studies'. The Eurasian journal of medicine, 43(2), 109–114. • Schoenfeld, B. (2011). 'Does cardio after an overnight fast maximize fat loss?'. Strength & Conditioning Journal, 33(1), 23–25. • Bellini, A. et al (2022). 'The Effects of Postprandial Walking on the Glucose Response after Meals with Different Characteristics'. Nutrients, 14(5), 1080. • Mahindru, A. et al (2023). 'Role of Physical Activity on Mental Health and Well-Being: A Review'. Cureus, 15(1), e33475. • Copeland, J. L. et al (2002). 'Hormonal responses to endurance and resistance exercise in females aged 19-69 years'. The journals of gerontology. Series A, Biological sciences and medical sciences, 57(4), B158–B165. • Varghese, S. et al (2024). 'Physical Exercise and the Gut Microbiome: A Bidirectional Relationship Influencing Health and Performance'. Nutrients, 16(21), 3663. • Noetel, M. et al (2024). 'Effect of exercise for depression: systematic review and network meta-analysis of randomised controlled trials'. BMJ 2024; 384 :e075847 • Fricke, A. et al (2021). 'Mini-Trampoline Jumping as an Exercise Intervention in Postmenopausal Women to Improve Women Specific Health Risk Factors'. International journal of preventive medicine, 12, 10.
184–94 ZOE. Going to bed earlier may prevent serious disease, ZOE study shows. • Baker, F. C. et al (2018). 'Sleep and sleep disorders

in the menopausal transition'. Sleep medicine clinics, 13(3), 443–456.
195–205 Lee, I. et al (2017). 'Increased risk of disordered eating in polycystic ovary syndrome'. Fertility and sterility, 107(3), 796–802. • Hsu, T. W. et al. (2024). 'Suicide attempts after a diagnosis of polycystic ovary syndrome: a cohort study'. Annals of internal medicine, 177(3), 335–342. • Laganà, A. S. et al. (2017). 'Anxiety and depression in patients with endometriosis: impact and management challenges'. International journal of women's health, 323–330 • Freeman, E. W. (2010). 'Associations of depression with the transition to menopause'. Menopause, 17(4), 823–827. • Lawrence, S. et al (2024). 'Post traumatic stress disorder associated hypothalamic-pituitary-adrenal axis dysregulation and physical illness'. Brain, Behavior, & Immunity-Health, 100849. • Kundakovic, M. et al (2022). 'Sex hormone fluctuation and increased female risk for depression and anxiety disorders: from clinical evidence to molecular mechanisms'. Frontiers in neuroendocrinology, 66, 101010. • Vitale, S. G. et al (2017). 'The impact of lifestyle, diet, and psychological stress on female fertility'. Oman Medical Journal, 32(5), 443. • Keyes, K. M.(2019). 'Is there a recent epidemic of women's drinking? A critical review of national studies'. Alcoholism: clinical and experimental research, 43(7), 1344–1359. • Cregg, D. R. et al (2023). 'Healing through helping: An experimental investigation of kindness, social activities, and reappraisal as well-being interventions'. The Journal of Positive Psychology, 18(6), 924–941. • Laranjeira, C.et al (2022). 'Hope and optimism as an opportunity to improve the "positive mental health" demand'. Frontiers in Psychology, 13, 827320. • CDC.gov. Social Connection. • Fryburg, D. A. (2022). 'Kindness as a stress reduction–health promotion intervention: a review of the psychobiology of caring'. American journal of lifestyle medicine, 16(1), 89–100.

Index

AUTHOR ACKNOWLEDGEMENTS

Thank you to my incredible team at DK, led by Zara Anvari, for your trust, talent, and support. To my editors, Amy Slack and Zoë Jellicoe, and designers, Barbara Zuniga and Eloise Myatt – you have brought my book to life so beautifully. Thank you to Silvia Dembner and Issy Panay. Thank you also to Arielle Steele for your editorial support.

Valeria Huerta, my agent – thank you for your belief in me, your kindness, and for finding the perfect home for my book. To my PR guru and co-pilot Aish Shah – I couldn't imagine this journey without you (or the voice notes).

To my children, Otis and Dusty – the apples of my eye and the thorns in my circadian rhythm's side. Thank you for being especially wonderful while I wrote this book – I love you. To my husband, Ben – as you often remind me, where would I be without you? Thank you for your love, unwavering support, and ability to make me laugh when I need it most.

Mum and Dad – I'm so grateful for your love, inspiring work ethic, and generosity as parents. Thank you for everything. Laura, my big sister – thank you, along with James, Lochie, and Christie, for always being there for me. Apple Nanny & Grandad and Bubbles Nanny & Grandad – I know how proud you would be. Thank you to all the Smith, Hope, Alderson, and Johnson family members.

To my precious friends, you know who you are. I cherish your love and support.

Thank you to the inspirational teachers in my life, particularly Mr and Mrs Kelley and Mr Gifford at Queenswood.

To my Design Bridge family, who taught me the power of storytelling, especially Dave Annetts and Claire Robertshaw – thank you for letting me follow my dream of studying nutrition while still working for you.

To my clients and members of the Positive Method club, past and present – thank you. I have the best job in the world.

And finally, to you, dear reader – thank you. May this book bring you health and happiness.

PUBLISHER ACKNOWLEDGEMENTS

DK would like to thank Phil Hunt for proofreading, Vanessa Bird for indexing, and Athena Stacy for editorial support. Thank you to Hannah Alderson for her use of her image on p224.

DK | Penguin Random House
[RED]

Senior Acquisitions Editor Zara Anvari
Acquisitions Editor Amy Slack
Senior Designer Barbara Zuniga
Sales Material & Jackets Coordinator Emily Cannings
Senior Production Editor Tony Phipps
Senior Production Controller Luca Bazzoli
Senior Picture Researcher Aditya Katyal
DTP and Design Co-ordinator Heather Blagden
Art Director Maxine Pedliham
Publishing Director Stephanie Jackson

Design Evi-O.Studio | Eloise Myatt
Editorial Zoë Jellicoe

First published in Great Britain in 2025 by
Dorling Kindersley Limited
20 Vauxhall Bridge Road,
London SW1V 2SA

The authorised representative in the EEA is
Dorling Kindersley Verlag GmbH. Arnulfstr. 124,
80636 Munich, Germany

A CIP catalogue record for this book
is available from the British Library.
ISBN: 978-0-2417-3392-9

Printed and bound in Slovakia

www.dk.com

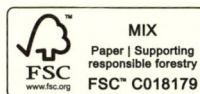

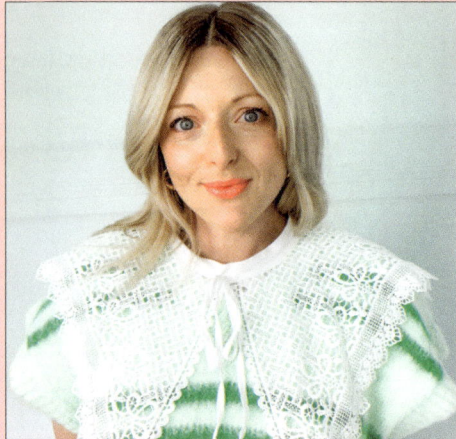

Hannah Alderson is a BANT-registered nutritionist who is on a mission to empower women, bridging the gap between flourishing hormones and overall wellbeing. She trained at the College of Naturopathic Medicine before furthering her studies with The Institute of Functional Medicine. She is a certified practitioner in eating disorders, a member of The British Menopause Society, and serves on the medical advisory board for the PCOSAA.

Drawing on her professional expertise and her own personal experience with PCOS and endometriosis, after qualifying Hannah set up her own global online private practice in 2018, through which she has transformed the lives of hundreds of clients. She has also launched The Positive Method Club, an online membership platform sharing guidance on hormone health and wellbeing.

Hannah can be found online at hannahalderson.com, or on Instagram @hannahaldersonnutrition.